CYTOLOGY
OF BONE TUMOURS

CYTOLOGY OF BONE TUMOURS

a colour atlas with text

N.G. Sanerkin MD, FRCPE
Consultant in Osteo-articular Pathology,
Bristol and Bath Health Districts and the South Western Region
Hon. Secretary, Bristol Bone Tumour Registry

and **G.M. Jeffree** BSc, PhD
Research Scientist,
Department of Osteo-articular Pathology, Bristol

J. B. Lippincott
Philadelphia · Toronto

ISBN 0-397-50523-X
Library of Congress Catalog Card Number 80-83508

PRINTED IN GREAT BRITAIN

PREFACE

The Bristol Bone Tumour Registry has been engaged in the study of bone tumours since its foundation in 1946 and its associated laboratory has functioned as a research and diagnostic centre devoted to the investigation and understanding of all aspects of bone tumours.

Two important developments have helped broaden its scope and diagnostic expertise. One has been the introduction and investigation of histochemical techniques since 1960, and one of us (G.M.J.) has been mainly engaged in this field. This work established the value of histochemistry in the precise diagnosis of some bone tumours, and we now know that routine histology, unaided by histochemistry, can sometimes lead to erroneous diagnosis, particularly in relation to osteosarcoma and its differentiation from fibrosarcoma, chondrosarcoma and anaplastic sarcomas. Inevitably, disappointments have also been experienced in that histochemistry has not solved some of the problems in which it might conceivably have helped—for instance, in determining the primary site with metastatic carcinomas.

The other significant development has been the application of cytology in the bone tumour field since 1969. The laboratory's established expertise in histochemical techniques was easily extended to smeared preparations, so that the study of cytomorphology was fully complemented by cytochemistry. The facility of preparation of cytological smears, as compared with cryostat sections, inevitably led to the replacement of histochemistry by cytochemistry. Considerable experience in the cytology of bone tumours has now accumulated and cytodiagnosis has become an integral part of the laboratory's routine work.

Every tumour received here is subjected to initial comprehensive cytomorphological and cytochemical study, followed by cryostat and paraffin sections, so that the cytology and histology are always closely compared and correlated with one another. We regard these methods of study as complementary, and not exclusive of one another; each adds to the understanding and evaluation of the other.

The cytological material in this atlas has, in natural consequence, been presented and described in direct comparison with the corresponding histology, and we hope that the manner of presentation will enhance its usefulness. Indeed, we would like to regard this volume as a vehicle for the better understanding of the pathology of bone tumours, and not merely as an exposition of their cytological appearances.

For whom is the atlas intended? First, for specialist centres such as ours which are engaged in the intensive study of bone tumours. We know of no other centre in the United Kingdom where our techniques are routinely employed. We suspect that this may be largely true of many other countries. We hope to convince the bone tumour expert of the value and rationale of cytodiagnostic practice as applied in this laboratory, for we are convinced that it would materially assist him in his task.

Second, this atlas is for the practitioners of needle aspiration cytodiagnosis in general, and there is an increasing number of these. Despite our express preference for cytodiagnosis based on ample surgical biopsy material, needle aspiration cytology will continue to be practised in many medical centres and some of this work will naturally include bone tumours. Our perusal of the literature, including books and atlases on general cytodiagnosis, indicates that relatively limited attention has been devoted to the detailed cytology of bone tumours; the full range of cytomorphology is not given and cytochemistry is, for the most part, either ignored or marginally dealt with. We hope that the illustrations in this volume, with their explicit descriptions, will prove of assistance to needle aspiration cytodiagnosticians.

Third, this atlas is for general histopathologists. Specialist bone tumour centres are, and are likely to remain, relatively few and most bone tumour material will continue to be dealt with primarily by the general histopathologist. The difficulties and pitfalls that confront the expert bone tumour pathologist can be even more formidable for the general histopathologist who, relatively and absolutely, sees so few of these tumours. We feel that the cytological information presented in this volume can materially assist the general pathologist in his diagnostic role. There is an additional reason why cytological smears of bone tumours should, whenever possible, be prepared in a general histopathology laboratory. A specialized centre such as ours naturally undertakes a considerable volume of referral work, because the general histopathologist, when faced with a difficult or unusual bone tumour, will refer his histological sections to the bone tumour specialist. The expert so consulted may be severely hampered by the lack of cytological information if, as sometimes happens, histology alone does not suffice in resolving the diagnostic problem. Submission of cytological smears in addition to histological sections during the referral will provide the referee with the additional information he may need for the correct diagnosis.

Fourth, we have in mind the orthopaedic surgeon interested in bone tumours. We hope that the material presented in this volume will enhance his appreciation of bone tumours and the full scope of their pathological investigation. In particular, it should draw his attention to the optimal manner in which biopsy or other surgical material should be handled, because the orthopaedic surgeon must necessarily take the *first* and *essential* step to ensure optimal investigation by desisting from the universal practice of placing all excised tissue directly into formol-saline or other fixative. He should direct the sampled tumour tissue to his pathologist in the fresh *unfixed* state; alternatively, he should place a small but representative fraction of the excised tumour tissue into a thermos flask (in the manner described in the introductory chapter, p.13) for delivery to his own pathologist or, if the latter cannot undertake the cytological investigation, to a specialist centre where such study can be undertaken.

Finally, this atlas is for all practitioners in locations or situations with inadequate facilities or expertise for histological diagnosis. We are sadly aware that even in some relatively developed countries, in some if not all their hospitals, the quality of histological technique and of histopathological diagnosis may be less than adequate in relation to bone pathology. In such circumstances, a smear stained with Haematoxylin and Eosin can establish whether a given bone tumour is benign or malignant. This, after all, is the most vital single information that the clinician seeks in dealing with any given bone tumour. We believe that such information can be reliably given, in most cases, by a simple cytological smear.

A word about the illustrations in this atlas. The colour photomicrographs have been taken on Kodak photomicrography film with a Leitz orthoplan microscope. The histological illustrations are mostly at a magnification of $\times 192$ and the cytological illustrations at a magnification of $\times 480$. Departures from these magnifications have been made in some cases, particularly when a low-power view was selected to elicit the general configuration of a given histological section or cytological smear. It should be emphasized here that low-power scanning is an important preliminary in the examination of cytological smears, as it is with histological sections.

June, 1980   N.G.S.   G.M.J.

ACKNOWLEDGEMENTS

Our thanks are due to the very numerous colleagues and various organizations who have supported the work of this laboratory and made it possible for us to prepare this volume.

We are greatly indebted to all past and present members of the Bristol Bone Tumour Registry whose constant guidance, collaboration and contributions have guided and sustained the work of this laboratory, in particular to Dr C.H.G. Price, who, until his retirement in 1975, was its director. Also to all the clinicians and pathologists in the West and South-West of England, and to many outside this region, who have facilitated our work by submitting fresh unfixed tumour material; likewise to all radiologists who have contributed X-ray material and advice. Without their conscientious and regular co-operation, the material on which this volume is based would not have been forthcoming. They are far too numerous to mention individually, but our gratitude to them is immense.

Until 1975, when this laboratory was taken over by the National Health Service, it was supported and maintained by grants from the Cancer Research Campaign. Since 1975 our research activities have been generously supported by the Dr Hadwen Trust. The Cancer Research Committee of the University of Bristol has always given moral and financial support to the laboratory. Highly appreciated financial contributions towards our research work have been made for many years by the pupils of St Mary Redcliffe and Temple School, Bristol.

We would like to record our appreciation and thanks to our technical staff, Mr B. Sims, Mr P.J. Hall and Mr A. Wilson, who have expertly and painstakingly carried out the technical work involved, helped with the photographic work and contributed the appendix on Technical Methods. We would like to thank Mrs J.E. Nutt for secretarial assistance.

CONTENTS

Chapter 1

Introduction

HISTORICAL

Non-exfoliative cytology

The subject matter of this volume is the non-exfoliative cytology of bone tumours and, to a lesser extent, of non-neoplastic lesions of the bones, and its correlation with the histopathology of these conditions.

Exfoliative cytology has only a small role to play in bone tumour work and any details of its historical background or application would be inappropriate in this introduction.

Non-exfoliative cytology was first applied some 50 years ago by Dudgeon and his associates (Dudgeon and Patrick, 1927; Dudgeon and Barrett, 1934), through the preparation of smears from surgically excised tumours. The cut surface of the excised tumour was scraped with a scalpel and the 'juice' so obtained spread on slides, fixed in Schaudinn's solution and stained with Haematoxylin and Eosin. Although their method admirably demonstrated the fine details of cell structure, it did not gain popularity in general pathological practice. The reason for this neglect is perhaps not difficult to understand. The surgical specimen from which such smears were made would soon be processed for histological sections, on which a diagnosis would be established in a day or two at the most. If an urgent opinion was required, then rapid frozen sections would be made.

The impetus for the more extensive use of non-exfoliative cytology came with the development and application of the needle biopsy technique, whereby material for cytological smears was obtained from deep-seated lesions. Shortly after Dudgeon's cytological work on surgically excised tissues, the application of needle aspiration in cytological diagnosis was reported (Martin and Ellis, 1930; Stewart, 1933), which also combined histology by paraffin-embedding fragments of tumour obtained by this procedure. Later, needle aspiration cytology was extensively applied and popularized by many others, including Cardozo (1954), Berg (1961), Zajicek (1965, 1974) and Söderström (1966).

Non-exfoliative cytology by the needle aspiration technique was applied more widely to bone tumours by Coley et al. (1931) and later by Snyder and Coley (1945), Schajowicz (1955), Schajowicz and Derqui (1968), Hajdu and Melamed (1971), Stormby and Akerman (1973), Hajdu and Hajdu (1976), Akerman et al. (1976), Thommesen and Frederiksen (1976) and Schajowicz and Hokama (1976). In most of these studies only a limited range of staining techniques was used. Hajdu and Hajdu (1976) devote a chapter to malignant bone tumours in their book on the cytopathology of sarcomas, based mainly on aspiration biopsy material and exfoliative smears but also including imprints from some excised tumours. Their account is necessarily limited in extent. Likewise, an even more limited chapter on bone tumour cytology is presented in Cardozo's atlas (1975). Salzer-Kuntschik (1976) gave a brief account of the cytomorphology and cytochemistry of bone tumours, based on imprints of surgically excised material.

In Bristol, non-exfoliative cytology of bone tumours has been studied in smears prepared from surgically excised tissues. The value of cytological smears in the diagnosis and understanding of bone tumours soon became abundantly evident, and the enzyme techniques which had formerly been applied to cryostat sections were soon devoted to cytological smears, so that cytochemistry has now largely supplanted histochemistry in our routine diagnostic practice.

Cytochemistry

The techniques applied for the demonstration of enzymes in cytological preparations do not differ from those applied to histological sections. As we have already mentioned, the cytochemical techniques used in our work were originally introduced and applied here in enzyme histochemistry (Jeffree and Price, 1965). Because enzyme histochemistry techniques were originally developed for histological sections, the following historical account necessarily relates to enzyme histochemistry.

Robison (1923) reported high phosphatase activity in young bones and ossifying cartilage. Further investigation showed optimal activity between pH 8·4 and 9·4 (Robison and Soames, 1924). This alkaline phosphatase was the first enzyme to be demonstrated histochemically, and independently, by Gomori (1939) and Takamatsu (1939), and its high activity in ossifying cartilage and embryonic perichondrium was reported at this time (Gomori, 1939). Similar high activity in osteosarcoma was demonstrated by Gomori's metal-substitution method shortly after this, in fowl osteosarcoma by Kabat and Furth (1941) and in human osteosarcoma by Gomori (1946). These observations were later confirmed with a variety of staining methods, including that of Burstone (1958a), who demonstrated high activity of alkaline phosphatase in both normal osteoblasts and the cells of an osteosarcoma of mouse.

Gomori (1946) also recorded intense alkaline phosphatase activity in the cells of Ewing's tumour, in contrast to those of other tumours of rather similar morphology, but this finding was not confirmed by Schajowicz and Cabrini (1954) who, using Gomori's technique, were unable to demonstrate alkaline phosphatase in this tumour, except in the blood vessels. In this laboratory, using the method of Burstone (1958a), alkaline phosphatase has only occasionally been found in the cells of Ewing's tumour; indeed these are more often negative (Jeffree, 1974).

The presence of alkaline phosphatase in the endothelium of small arterioles and capillaries has been reported by a number of workers, from Gomori (1939) onwards (Kabat and Furth, 1941; Greep et al., 1948; Schajowicz and Cabrini, 1954; Burstone, 1958a; Monis and Rutenburg, 1960; Romanul and Bannister, 1962). Endothelial cells may often be seen in cytological preparations, and they form a useful positive control for alkaline phosphatase staining where the lesional cells themselves are negative.

Alkaline phosphatase may be visualized in fibroblasts in a variety of conditions— in healing wounds (Fell and Danielli, 1943), in the fibrous stroma of carcinomas (Monis and Rutenburg, 1960) and to varying degrees in non-ossifying fibroma (Jeffree, 1972), but reports on fibrosarcoma are almost entirely negative (Kabat and Furth, 1941; Jeffree, 1972). By contrast, Schajowicz and Cabrini (1954) found high activity in a specimen of fibrous dysplasia. This observation was confirmed by Changus (1957) who referred to the cells of this lesion as 'histochemical osteoblasts'.

Weak activity of the lysosomal enzyme acid phosphatase is almost ubiquitous, but high activity appears to be characteristic of phagocytic cells of various origins, as well as of a variety of secretory cells. Gomori (1946) found the most intense staining for this enzyme in the cells of prostatic carcinoma and in normal prostatic epithelium. He also noted activity in giant-cell tumours of bone. High activity in the multinucleate cells of this tumour and in normal osteoclasts has since been recorded many times with a variety of techniques (Pepler, 1958; Schajowicz and Cabrini, 1958; Burstone, 1959; Schajowicz, 1961).

The original metal deposition methods of Takamatsu (1939) and Gomori (1939, 1946) for alkaline and acid phosphatases are still, with minor modifications, in common use. They have the advantage of utilizing more or less natural substrates and of being demonstrable by electron microscopy, but bone itself is also stained, which is a limitation in this type of work. There is also a wide range of azo-dye techniques, based on the formation of insoluble dyes by coupling stable diazotates with the variously substituted naphthols liberated from their phosphate esters by enzyme activity. The earliest of these methods (Menten et al., 1944) utilized beta-naphthyl phosphate and freshly-diazotized beta-naphthylamine. Manheimer and Seligman (1949) used stable diazotates in a similar method, and the technique was further modified by the use, first, of sodium alpha-naphthyl phosphate, then of the phosphate esters of AS-Naphthol and its derivatives, culminating in the methods of Burstone (1958a,b) which are used in this laboratory.

The histochemical demonstration of beta-glucuronidase is of comparatively recent date. The post-coupling azo-dye method of Seligman et al. (1954) with 6-bromo-2-naphthyl-beta-glucuronidase as substrate was moderately satisfactory, but convenient simple methods of staining date from the use of Naphthol AS-BI-beta-glucuronide, which was used by Fishman (1964) in a post-coupling technique with Fast Dark Blue R; by Hayashi et al. (1964) with simultaneous coupling with freshly diazotized pararosanilin, and by Jeffree (1969) with simultaneous coupling with Bordeaux OL or Red-Violet LB salts. The latter method is in use in this laboratory.

Like acid phosphatase, beta-glucuronidase is largely a lysosomal enzyme and it has a rather similar distribution in phagocytic cells such as osteoclasts, the multinucleate cells of giant-cell tumour of bone, and both normal and neoplastic histiocytes. It is not, however, entirely lysosomal, nor necessarily present in the same lysosomes as those secreting acid phosphatase. It was reported by Fishman and Anlyan (1947) to be raised in neoplastic tissues, and high activity may often be seen in carcinomas, particularly carcinoma of the breast (Jeffree, 1969, 1974). In normal plasma cells there is moderately strong activity of this enzyme, but in myeloma cells it is generally intense, often in large bizarre globules, possibly associated with immunoglobulin production (Jeffree, 1974).

GENERAL PRINCIPLES OF CYTODIAGNOSIS

Intimate knowledge of the histology of normal and abnormal tissues is an essential prerequisite to the discriminant and intelligent practice of diagnostic cytology. Equally, detailed knowledge of the structure of normal and abnormal cells, as afforded by smeared preparations, provides an invaluable basis for the appreciation of histopathology, for histology relies on the recognition of cells and their arrangement and organization into tissues. In our own practice the cytomorphology and cytochemistry of bone lesions are studied in close and direct correlation with their histology, and such a comparison will form an essential purpose and basis of this volume. The general principles that underlie this comparison are set out below.

Normal histology and cytology
In normal tissues a state of balance exists in the regeneration and development of the constituent cells, so that the appearance and arrangement of the cells remain constant. The individual cell regenerates through mitosis, develops or differentiates into maturity and eventually undergoes senescence and dies. During this normal process it inevitably undergoes alterations in its nuclear and cytoplasmic size and appearance. Thus, any particular family of normal cells must have nuclear and cytoplasmic pleomorphism within a well-defined normal range intrinsic to that special group. This normal pleomorphism is clearly evident in the bone marrow, in which the progenitor cells, such as the haemocytoblast, myeloblast and proerythroblast, differ in their nuclear and cytoplasmic size and appearance from their differentiating and mature progeny. Similarly, in various epithelia a normal pleomorphism exists between the progenitor—basal or reserve—cells and the maturing, differentiated and senile cells. This is particularly obvious in the epidermis and the seminiferous tubules of the testis, but occurs to varying degrees in all epithelia. In the connective tissues the morphological differences between the juvenile cells—osteoblasts, fibroblasts, chondroblasts and lipoblasts—and the mature quiescent cells—osteocytes, fibrocytes, chondrocytes and lipocytes—are quite obvious. In all tissues, the progenitor cells tend to have large juvenile nuclei with nucleoli and may show mitoses, the frequency of which depends on the normal turnover of the particular tissue; their cytoplasm is as yet undifferentiated, and the nucleo-cytoplasmic ratio is high. With increasing maturity, the nucleus undergoes condensation of its chromatin, so that it becomes smaller and darker, and specific activity or differentiation becomes evident in the cytoplasm; for instance, differentiated glandular cells will show secretory activity, epidermal cells will keratinize, melanocytes will produce pigment, and various connective tissue cells will have manufactured interstitial matrix such as collagen, cartilage or bone.

Smears from normal tissues conform in their cellularity and cytomorphology to the normal range noted in histological sections. As far as the connective tissues are concerned, it is practically impossible to obtain smears from normal bone (as distinct from bone-marrow), cartilage, collagenous tissue or adipose tissue. Any attempt to smear cancellous bone will yield a smear of the marrow elements; compact cortical bone cannot be smeared at all. Only scanty cells can be expressed from normal cartilage, and then only if the cartilage is forcibly crushed between the forceps. Fibrocytes are firmly entrapped in mature collagen, and only a random cell will be dislodged in any attempt to smear such tissue. An attempt to smear normal adipose tissue will rupture most of the adipocytes, leaving small compact condensed nuclei in a mass of discharged fat. For this reason, our experience of the cytology of non-neoplastic connective tissues largely relates to reactive proliferations.

Histology and cytology of reactive proliferations
In reactive proliferations, such as repair processes and hyperplasias, the tissue involved undergoes normal accelerated regeneration of its progenitor cells, so that

the relative numbers of the juvenile cells greatly increase in proportion to the more mature or differentiated cells, particularly at the earlier stages of proliferation. Increased mitotic activity is seen as a reflection of this accelerated regenerative process.

Smears from regenerative proliferations show a relative predominance of normal active juvenile cells, with a relatively high mitotic activity. In the connective tissues, the best examples of reactive proliferation are seen with fracture callus and myositis ossificans in their earlier stages (*see* Chapter 2, pages 19–26), in which reactive young fibroblasts, osteoblasts and sometimes chondroblasts are found.

Histology and cytology of inflammatory reactions
In inflammatory reactions the host tissue undergoes hyperaemia, oedema and infiltration by inflammatory cells of various types (polymorphonuclear leucocytes, lymphocytes, plasma cells, eosinophils, histiocytes) according to the nature and duration of the particular inflammatory process involved. In most inflammatory reactions, the host tissue suffers variable disruption, degeneration and necrosis, and eventually undergoes some degree of reactive and reparative change.

Smears from inflammatory lesions will reflect the nature of the inflammatory process which is present. Acute inflammatory reactions produce a smear rich in polymorphonuclear leucocytes in various stages of degeneration. In subacute inflammatory processes, in addition to the granulocytes, there are numbers of histiocytes, many of which will contain engulfed pus cells and cellular debris. In non-specific chronic inflammatory reactions there will be a predominance of lymphocytes and plasma cells, with a variable admixture of polymorphonuclear leucocytes and histiocytes. In granulomatous inflammations, such as tuberculosis, there are abundant histiocytes, including multinucleate Langhans-type giant cells, necrotic debris and a variable admixture of lymphocytes and polymorphonuclears.

Histology and cytology of metaplastic lesions
In metaplasias, the development of a given tissue deviates from that normally expected and, instead, conforms to that of some other tissue. Metaplasia may occur in both non-neoplastic and neoplastic states. For instance, squamous and 'intestinal' metaplasia may occur in non-neoplastic glandular epithelia, and non-neoplastic connective tissues may undergo myxoid metaplasia, as in the formation of 'ganglia', as well as chondroid or osteoid metaplasia, as in synovial chondromatosis and myositis ossificans. In malignant conditions, squamous metaplasia may occur in adenocarcinomas, e.g. of the endometrium, gallbladder and colon, and in transitional-cell carcinomas, e.g. of the bladder, and examples of metaplasia are seen in sarcomas, for instance chondroblastic metaplasia in osteosarcoma, myxoid change in liposarcomas, fibrosarcomas and rhabdomyosarcomas.

Metaplasia may be recognized in cytological smears in certain conditions. The osteoblasts seen in smears of myositis ossificans develop by metaplasia of fibroblasts and their precursors. In smears from osteosarcoma malignant osteoblasts may manifest some chondroblastic metaplasia. Squamous metaplasia, as evidenced by the presence of keratinized squamous cells, can be found in smears from some urothelial carcinomas.

Histology and cytology of benign neoplasms
In benign neoplasms the cellular proliferation approximates to a considerable degree in its cytomorphology and maturity to the normal tissues of origin; likewise

the arrangement and organization of the constituent cells conform more closely to the normal tissues than is the case with malignant tumours. The rate of growth and mitotic activity are relatively low. The tumour does not show evidence of invasive activity; in particular blood and lymphatic channels are not permeated by tumour.

In smears from benign neoplasms the cell morphology, whilst departing from the normal, generally approximates more to the normal cell than to its malignant counterpart. In particular, the nuclei are smaller than those of malignant cells, more uniform in size and have a more mature chromatin structure. Slight, if any, mitotic activity is found and any mitoses are of normal type.

Histology and cytology of malignant neoplasms

In malignant neoplasms there is uncontrolled proliferation by abnormal cells which significantly differ in their appearance from the normal cell, and the abnormal cells are arranged or organized in a manner which significantly departs from the normal. In histological sections, the uncontrolled proliferation is associated with infiltration of the adjoining tissues and permeation of the lumina of lymphatic and blood vessels, attesting to the metastatic potential which is the hallmark of malignancy.

Apart from such manifestations as invasiveness and vascular permeation, the histological recognition of malignancy is based, to a large extent, on the abnormal appearance and arrangement of its constituent cells. The most striking alteration is in the nuclear appearance. The nuclei are large and primitive, usually show significant variations in size, giant or multiple nuclei may be present, there is a high mitotic rate, and abnormal mitoses may occur. The nuclear chromatin is abnormal in appearance and distribution, with coarse irregular clumping or diffuse hyperchromasia; the nucleoli are usually prominent, may be irregular or multiple. The malignant cells may show no cytoplasmic differentiation whatsoever, so that the tumour appears undifferentiated or anaplastic. Often, however, some degree of differentiation can be found, but the differentiation never conforms to that of the corresponding normal cells and remains as a caricature of the latter.

Malignant cells, like normal cells, may undergo maturity and senescence, the clearest evidence of which is the condensation of the nuclear chromatin and a corresponding reduction in the nuclear size as compared with the younger tumour cells. Scattered necrotic cells are frequently seen in malignant tumours; this is distinct from the more extensive focal or confluent tissue necrosis which is found within the tumour as a result of interference with its blood supply.

All the cellular abnormalities which are recognized in histological sections of malignant tumours can be observed in clearer detail in cytological smears. Recognition of malignancy is by far the most important function in cytodiagnosis, and the following criteria apply.

1. Cell population

A high density of cells is usually found in smears from malignant tumours. There are exceptions to this: for instance, fibrosarcomas with collagenization yield scanty smears, likewise scirrhous metastatic carcinomas in which the bulk of the lesion may be formed by fibrous tissue. Furthermore, high cell density can usually be found in non-sarcomatous bone lesions such as conventional giant-cell tumour, non-ossifying fibroma and chondroblastoma.

Relatively high cellularity is of particular significance in smears from cartilage tumours. Chondrosarcomas are comparatively easy to smear and yield relatively abundant cells, whereas benign cartilage lesions are difficult to smear and yield scanty cell populations.

2. Variations in cell size and shape

Anisocytosis is a common feature of smears from malignant tumours, and is particularly well marked in osteosarcomas in which giant tumour cells often abound. This is not, however, true of all malignant tumours which may be met in bone. For instance, some leukaemic deposits, lymphosarcomas, Ewing's tumour and certain metastatic carcinomas may show little or no anisocytosis.

Furthermore, anisocytosis may be a normal feature of certain benign bone lesions which intrinsically contain a variable admixture of cells of different shape and size; conventional giant-cell tumour, non-ossifying fibroma, chondromyxoid fibroma and chondroblastoma contain an admixture of osteoclasts, fusiform cells and rounded or oval cells. The anisocytosis in such lesions is readily recognized as a characteristic feature of the particular lesion and by itself does not raise any suspicion of malignancy.

3. Presence of necrotic cells

Smears from malignant tumours often contain scattered degenerate and necrotic cells.

4. Nuclear abnormalities

These form the most important criteria for the cytological diagnosis of malignancy:
- a. *Nuclear size:* The nuclei of malignant cells are larger than those of the corresponding cell in normal tissues, reactive proliferations and benign neoplasms. Nuclear size, however, can be difficult to judge in any individual smear when that smear is viewed without direct comparison with the normal, reactive or benign neoplastic cell. In some of the subsequent chapters, outline drawings will be given comparing the nuclear size in malignant and non-malignant cells.
- b. *Nuclear pleomorphism:* Anisokaryosis is a striking and very important feature of most malignant neoplasms, and this is a particularly prominent characteristic of osteosarcomas in which huge polyploid nuclei are common. Nuclear pleomorphism is immediately and easily recognizable in smears in which it is present.

  Nevertheless, nuclear pleomorphism is not a universal feature of all malignant tumours; for instance, Ewing's tumour and some metastatic adenocarcinomas may show relatively uniform nuclear size.
- c. *Multiple nuclei:* In addition to huge polyploid single nuclei, multiple nuclei—the end-result of abnormal multipolar mitosis in polyploid nuclei— can be found in smears from malignant tumours, particularly of sarcomas. Cells with giant single nuclei or with multiple nuclei are perforce giant-sized cells, i.e. tumour giant-cells. Multinucleate giant tumour cells are readily distinguishable from osteoclasts which may be found, either incidentally or as part of the lesion, in many smears from bone lesions. The nuclei of osteoclasts are of normal size and appearance, whereas the nuclei of multinucleate tumour giant-cells are large and hyperchromatic.

  The presence of multiple nuclei is an extremely helpful feature in the cytological differentiation of low-grade or medium-grade chondrosarcomas from benign cartilage tumours.

d. *Nuclear chromatin structure:* The nuclear chromatin of malignant cells shows abnormalities in its structure and distribution when compared with non-malignant cells of similar origin.

Hyperchromasia is a frequent finding in malignant cells, and refers to uniformly heavy dark staining of the nucleus. Implicitly the hyperchromatic nucleus is, at the same time, a large primitive nucleus. Dark nuclei are also a feature of mature and especially of senescent cells in which the nuclear chromatin condenses and the nuclear size shrinks. The malignant cell with a large dark *hyperchromatic* nucleus will show other features of its character; it will have prominent nucleoli, a high nucleo-cytoplasmic ratio, and often lack differentiation of its cytoplasm. The mature or senescent cell with a small dark *condensed* nucleus will have no nucleoli, its nucleo-cytoplasmic ratio will be low, and the cytoplasm may show evidence of differentiation. It should be stressed that condensation of nuclear chromatin will occur in all senescent cells, whether these are non-malignant or malignant. Nevertheless, the condensed nucleus of a senescent malignant cell will be *larger* than the condensed nucleus of a senescent non-malignant cell.

In some cases, the excess chromatin in the nucleus of the malignant cell may be arranged irregularly, rather than uniformly, producing a coarsely clumped pattern.

Hyperchromasia and coarse clumping of chromatin are not invariably present in the nuclei of all malignant tumours; in some tumours the chromatin may be dispersed as fine sharply outlined granules, producing a stippled pattern. For instance, chondrosarcoma and chondroblastic osteosarcoma may have such 'open' stippled nuclei; so may reticulosarcoma and some adenocarcinomas. Stippled nuclear chromatin is also a frequent feature of juvenile non-neoplastic cells, but in the malignant cell the nucleus is larger than in the corresponding reactive normal cell.

e. *Nucleoli:* Malignant cells tend to have nucleolar abnormalities when compared with normal cells at comparable stages of maturity; indeed, nucleoli may persist in relatively mature malignant cells. The nucleoli may be exceptionally large, numerous or of irregular shape.

f. *Mitotic activity:* Mitoses are frequent in malignant smears; they can be regularly and easily found in most cases. This observation does not apply to low-grade or medium-grade chondrosarcomas, in which it is exceptional to find mitoses.

It should be remembered that mitoses can be frequent in reactive proliferations such as fracture callus and myositis ossificans; they merely indicate a rapid rate of regeneration in the sampled tissue. Conventional giant-cell tumour invariably shows fair numbers of mitoses in its stromal cells. Mitoses are infrequent in such non-malignant bone tumours as osteoblastoma, chondroblastoma, chondromyxoid fibroma and non-ossifying fibroma.

g. *Abnormal mitoses:* Abnormal mitoses, which may be tripolar or otherwise multipolar, can often be found in smears from malignant tumours. They are a reflection of the nuclear polyploidy of such tumours and a very good indication of malignancy.

It should be admitted that multipolar mitoses can sometimes be seen in normal cells, e.g. in megakaryocytes of normal or reactive bone-marrow. In practice, this is an extremely rare finding and never gives rise to any confusion, since the multipolar mitosis is recognizably in a normal cell in a normal marrow smear.

Differences between malignant cells of epithelial and connective tissue origin

The most important and reliable differences between carcinoma and sarcoma cells in cytological smears are:

a. The propensity of carcinoma cells to cluster or adhere to one another. It is infrequent, in a smear from a carcinoma, not to see small circumscribed clusters or well-defined 'Indian-file' rows of tumour cells.

b. Carcinomas tend to show the cytoplasmic differentiation expected in epithelial cells, such as mucin secretion, keratinization or brush borders.

We have found nuclear differences between carcinomas and sarcomas inconstant and unreliable. As a general rule, sarcoma cells tend to have greater nuclear pleomorphism and coarser chromatin distribution than carcinoma cells, but we have learnt from experience not to devote too much attention to nuclear detail in deciding whether a given malignant smear is carcinomatous or sarcomatous.

SCOPE AND PURPOSE OF CYTOLOGY IN BONE TUMOUR WORK

Our experience in the cytodiagnosis of bone tumours has been based on non-exfoliative cytology, with an express preference for the open surgical biopsy rather than the needle aspiration biopsy. We do not use cytology as an alternative to histology but specifically aim at broadening our sources of pathological information by using cytology, both cytomorphology and cytochemistry, as an adjunct to histology.

In bone tumour work there can be little scope for exfoliative cytology. Hajdu and Hajdu (1976) illustrate examples in which cells from metastatic osteosarcoma and chondrosarcoma have been identified in the sputum or pleural fluid. It is also conceivable that, rarely, it might be possible to examine the synovial fluid for malignant cells when a tumour encroaches the joint space whether by direct extension or through a pathological fracture.

The advantages and limitations of needle aspiration cytology, as compared with cytological preparations from ample surgical biopsy material, will be discussed below.

Needle aspiration cytology

Smears from needle aspiration biopsy can provide diagnostic information in tumours and non-neoplastic lesions of bone. Nevertheless, there are various limitations to the use of needle biopsy techniques in bone tumour work.

1. Not all bone lesions are readily accessible to needle aspiration biopsy, many being endosteal.

2. There is always the possibility that needle aspiration may yield an unrepresentative sample, for instance of reactive tissue from beyond the margins of the lesion, from an area which is completely necrotic, or only blood may be aspirated. The structure of a tumour may vary in different parts; for instance, a chondrosarcoma may harbour areas indistinguishable from a chondroma, and a blind sample from such banal areas may lead to an erroneous diagnosis. These pitfalls and difficulties may, indeed, be occasionally experienced even with generous open surgical biopsy, but skilled selective sampling is undoubtedly far superior to random blind aspiration of minimal lesional tissue.

3. In most cases a needle aspiration cytodiagnosis would have to be followed by open surgical biopsy for a variety of reasons:

  a. For histological confirmation of the cytological diagnosis. This may be possible with a wide-bore needle biopsy, as compared with the fine-needle aspiration biopsy, but even a cylinder of tissue from a wide-bore needle will probably be inadequate for proper assessment of a bone tumour.

  b. For detailed study of the structure of the tumour, including the identification of its invasive characteristics and any vascular permeation, an exercise which requires a generous sample of the tumour.

  c. To establish that the needle sample has, in fact, been representative of the lesion as a whole.

  d. Where cytology has provided only a broad or generic diagnosis, e.g. inflammatory, 'malignant round-cell tumour', cartilage tumour, to determine the precise categorization within that broad group.

4. Needle aspiration biopsy samples will provide relatively few smears for detailed and specialized study. In a major centre, a dozen smears may be required for various staining procedures and ample material would be advisable for cryostat and paraffin sections; further tissue would also be needed for tissue culture and E.M. studies.

Despite our preference for open surgical biopsy smears, there are occasions on which needle aspiration biopsy may be the first choice and may suffice for the definitive diagnosis, for instance:

  a. Destructive lesions in the spinal column, in which an open biopsy would necessitate fairly major surgery. A needle aspiration biopsy may suffice for the diagnosis of, say, metastatic carcinoma, plasma-cell myeloma or eosinophilic granuloma.

  b. In infants with clinically atypical osteomyelitis, which may sometimes raise suspicion of a malignant tumour, a needle aspiration smear may show a typical acute inflammatory exudate and thus circumvent the need for surgical exploration.

  c. In osteosarcomas with extra-osseous extension, a needle aspiration smear should provide a clear-cut confirmation of the diagnosis, so that the surgeon may proceed to perform the definitive operation without any open biopsy.

There is a further practical use for needle aspiration cytology which would apply in situations with limited laboratory facilities. In can be utilized in relatively underdeveloped areas, even without technical facilities for histological processing, where it should provide diagnostic information even in relatively inexperienced hands.

Cytological smears from open biopsy specimens

It is our practice to receive surgical material from bone tumours in the fresh unfixed state and to prepare immediate cytological smears. A relatively small fraction of the specimen, if necessary only a few millimetres in diameter, will usually suffice for the preparation of a dozen or so smears. The rest of the specimen is then apportioned for further investigations, including cryostat and paraffin sections as well as ultra-thin sections for electron microscopy.

To many general histopathologists, the need for cytological investigation might appear incongruous when adequate material has already been received for histology, including cryostat sections. There are several excellent reasons why cytological studies should be undertaken in these circumstances:

a. They permit very rapid diagnosis, always in a shorter period of time and, in most cases, far more confidently than is possible with cryostat sections when dealing with primary bone tumours. An urgent diagnosis as to whether the lesion is benign or malignant can be given in a matter of minutes, the time it takes to make a routine HE stain. An exact diagnosis of osteosarcoma can be made within 15–20 minutes, the time it takes to make an alkaline phosphatase preparation. Such a firm diagnosis of osteosarcoma is possible even with samples in which the diagnosis would be impossible with paraffin sections, i.e. in the absence of demonstrable tumour osteoid.

b. They enable the pathologist to study the fine cytological detail of the lesional cells to a degree that is not possible with histological sections, whether in routine paraffin sections or in semi-thin sections after resin embedding. We have found from experience that an intimate familiarity with cytological detail derived from the study of smears, and the regular correlation of smears with histological sections, renders the appreciation and assessment of histological detail all the more satisfying and profitable.

c. A large number of smears can be prepared for special staining procedures designed to demonstrate both the cytomorphological and cytochemical features of individual lesional cells. The general distribution of enzymes in a given tissue can be observed in cryostat sections, but the identification of individual cell types is far less satisfactory with such sections.

The pathologist dealing with bone tumours relies on the thorough assessment of all available information—clinical, radiological and pathological—in arriving at the correct diagnosis. He regards cytology as an additional and valuable source of information, complementary to histology, and sees no particular virtue in dealing with minimal tumour samples obtained by needle aspiration biopsy.

Limited information, through neglect of one or more of the available sources, can lead to erroneous conclusions. For instance, it has been known at this Registry for a correct X-ray diagnosis to have been made of osteosarcoma when the histology was interpreted by experienced pathologists as some other malignant tumour, such as malignant giant-cell tumour; cytomorphological and cytochemical information, if it had been available at the initial biopsy, would have helped establish a pathological diagnosis of osteosarcoma. Florid fracture callus and myositis ossificans in its early stages can, particularly with limited biopsy material, be difficult to differentiate from osteosarcoma on histology alone, whereas cytological smears would leave no possible doubt as to their reactive nature. The histological diagnosis of cartilage tumours, particularly in discriminating between chondroma and low-grade chondrosarcoma at one extreme, and between high-grade chondrosarcoma and chondroblastic osteosarcoma at the other extreme, has always been difficult and sometimes fallible. It has been known even for the most experienced bone tumour pathologist to make a histological diagnosis of benign chondroma in a cartilage tumour which eventually leaves no doubt of its true nature by metastasizing. The current histological criteria for the diagnosis of chondrosarcoma are mainly based on the cytological appearance, and particularly on the nuclear structure, of the individual tumour cells *as observed in tissue sections*. It is abundantly obvious that cytological detail can best be observed in smears, hence the importance of cytology in dealing with cartilage tumours cannot be over-emphasized. In cartilage tumours, it is important that the cytological smears should be prepared from the most suspicious, i.e. the most cellular looking, areas of the excised tumour tissue. A large biopsy specimen is more likely to provide the opportunity for such selective sampling in the preparation of cytological smears.

The general histopathologist might also enquire why we should prefer cytologi-cal smears to cryostat sections for rapid diagnosis or for enzyme studies:

1. We have found cytology far more reliable than cryostat sections for the rapid diagnosis of primary malignant tumours of bone. In our experience cryostat sections are not always satisfactory for the diagnosis of sarcomas and we suspect this might be equally true, perhaps more so, of general histopathologists. We have known, for intance, for a diagnosis of Histiocytosis X to have been made on cryostat sections of a pleomorphic osteosarcoma, because of an associated over-abundance of eosinophils, whereas cytology would have established the correct diagnosis.

2. Cryostat sections may not always be convenient or practicable, for instance with—

    a. Fragments of tissue which are partly osseous. Cryostat sections from such material would be difficult, even in experienced hands with specialized equipment, whereas tumour cells can always be scraped or expressed from such material.

    b. Cartilage tumours, in which one relies heavily on cytological detail. Cryostat sections are unsuitable for fine cytological detail, whereas smears are optimal for this purpose.

    c. With limited biopsy material, adequate tissue may not be available for both cryostat and paraffin sections. Paraffin sections can, of course, be prepared from tissue already used for cryostat sections but paraffin sections from tissues which have previously been frozen are often imperfect. Smears can be prepared even from the most limited biopsy material and still leave the bulk of the tissue available for paraffin sections.

We can give one example in which we have had a needle biopsy cylinder less than 2 mm thick and about 1 cm long from the extra-osseous extension of an osteosarcoma. A 2 mm long fraction of this was smeared on several slides and a perfectly obvious diagnosis of osteosarcoma was made on the basis of a sarcomatous smear which was strongly alkaline phosphatase positive. The remaining 8 mm length was processed for paraffin sections, but the histology was adequate only for the diagnosis of malignancy and not of osteosarcoma.

Cryostat sections are indeed employed in this laboratory, but there are specific reasons for their use in addition to smears:

1. Cryostat sections reveal the tissue structure of the tumour, which smears obviously do not. On occasions, a smear from an anaplastic metastatic carcinoma may fail to establish the diagnosis but instead simulate a 'malignant round-cell tumour'. Cryostat sections easily resolve the problem by demonstrating the characteristic parcelled or trabecular arrangement which most carcinomas display histologically. Likewise, a childhood sarcoma, such as alveolar or embryonal rhabdomyosarcoma, can yield a smear which is predominantly round-celled so that it may simulate a 'malignant round-cell tumour'; cryostat sections will clearly demonstrate the alveolar pattern of alveolar rhabdomyosarcoma and indicate the correct diagnosis.

2. Smears from malignant tumours may contain numbers of lipid-laden tumour cells and one cannot always be certain whether these are an intrinsic feature of the tumour or the result of degenerative change. Cryostat sections, essential for the demonstration of lipid in tissues, help display the distribution of such lipid-containing tumour cells. When due to degeneration such cells often border foci of

necrosis, whereas in liposarcoma they are found in perfectly viable areas.

3. Cryostat sections will demonstrate the geographical distribution of various enzymes in the tissue as a whole; this is not possible with smears.

APPLICATION OF CYTOLOGICAL TECHNIQUES IN BONE TUMOUR WORK

Delivery of specimens

As already mentioned, we aim to receive surgical material from bone tumours in the unfixed fresh state, whether or not an urgent diagnosis is required. It is naturally desirable to minimize the time interval between the excision and examination of such material, and urgent specimens are of necessity immediately delivered. Any specimen which cannot be delivered without delay should be kept in a refrigerator until delivery. Minute fragments will suffer from desiccation whether kept refrigerated or not, with serious deterioration of both cytological and histological detail. Minute samples should therefore be delivered promptly or else kept moist by wrapping in absorbent cloth or paper soaked in normal saline. Specimens submitted from other centres can be sent by post or rail provided the sample is packaged in a sealed plastic envelope and placed in a thermos flask with the addition of ice to keep the flask cool.

Experience has shown that an overnight delay in delivery will not make any significant difference to the cytomorphology of the cells or cause any detectable deterioration in their enzymatic properties, certainly so far as acid and alkaline phosphatases are concerned. We have on occasion received unrefrigerated amputation specimens from outside the United Kingdom, wrapped in formalin-soaked cloth, in which the intra-osseous tumour was entirely unfixed; from such specimens, after several days' delay in delivery, we have obtained smears of adequate diagnostic quality, with good enzyme preservation.

Preparation of smears

A *good* smear is an essential preliminary to satisfactory cytodiagnostic work. The occasional smear prepared in the operating theatre by the surgeon is, more often than not, of poor quality. In our laboratory, the pathologist himself carefully and selectively prepares the smears. Excess fluid, particularly blood, delays the drying of the smears and so prevents the flattening of the smeared cells. For this reason, it is desirable to remove excess blood from the tissue fragment by daubing it on a paper towel. The fragment is then held between the tips of a dissecting forceps, pressed on a clean microscopic slide and moved across its surface with a circular or elliptical motion. The amount of pressure required will depend on the texture and cohesiveness of the particular tissue. With osteosarcomas, 'malignant round-cell tumours', giant-cell tumours, non-ossifying fibromas, inflammatory lesions and cellular metastatic carcinomas a light touch only is required during smearing. With sclerotic tumours, such as some fibrosarcomas and scirrhous metastatic carcinomas, and with cartilage tumours with well-formed matrix, considerable pressure may be necessary. Such specimens are best squeezed firmly or crushed between the tips of the forceps; the aim is to squeeze or force out a proportion of the cells from the entrapping matrix with the accompanying tissue fluid and spread the expressed material across the slide. The cell population derived from such fibrous or cartilaginous material will perforce be relatively scanty, but sufficient cells will be smeared for satisfactory assessment. It must be stressed that there is no particular virtue in being over-gentle in the smearing process, for no amount of rough handling will damage more than a proportion of the smeared cells.

The total amount of tissue used in making a dozen smears need not be more than a few millimetres in diameter. Whenever possible, it is preferable not to use a given aliquot of tissue for more than three or four smears; it is better to divide it into three or four separate fractions and to use these in turn to make the dozen smears. The actual size of the tissue used for smears will, in practice, depend on the amount of tissue submitted for examination. With most biopsy material, there will be no need to reduce the amount of tissue used to the barest minimum.

With most samples, provided excess surface blood and fluid has been daubed off, the smear dries off practically as soon as it is spread. If the drying process appears to be slow, it may be necessary to wave the slide rapidly in the air to speed up the drying process; we do not often have to resort to this latter exercise.

Staining of smears
The staining procedures used in our laboratory are given below. Of this list, a minimum of six stains—Haematoxylin and Eosin (HE), Taylor's blue, PAS, PAS-diastase and preparations for alkaline and acid phosphatase—are considered essential for bone tumour cytology.

1. *Haematoxylin and Eosin.* The air-dried smear must first be fixed in cold acetone, otherwise nuclear detail will be poor. After cold acetone fixation, the nuclear detail is excellent. Fixation in alcohol may be used as an alternative.

HE is the stain, above all other routine stains, which we prefer for diagnostic cytology. In exfoliative cytology, many centres employ a Papanicolaou staining procedure because most exfoliative cytologists have been trained on and deal with cervical smears. In needle aspiration cytology much of the pioneer work has been done with Romanowsky stains, such as Giemsa and Leishman, and these stains continue to be the mainstay of non-exfoliative cytodiagnosis in many centres.

We firmly favour HE for routine cytomorphological investigation of smears from bone tumours. Nuclear and cytoplasmic detail is quite admirably and consistently displayed by this method. Furthermore, the histopathologist uses HE routinely for staining paraffin sections, and in our work we constantly compare the cytomorphology of a given tumour with the histological appearances of that tumour. Only HE permits such a close correlation.

2. *Giemsa.* We have always included this in our staining procedures, if only because by historical precedent it has been employed by most non-exfoliative cytodiagnosticians. We have not, however, found it comparable in its practical usefulness to HE. The quality of staining is always uneven and inconstant, difficult to control and can be very poor indeed. On occasions, it will provide good results, for instance with tumours of the haemopoietic or lympho-histiocytic groups such as myelomatosis, leukaemias and some round-cell tumours; but all these can be stained perfectly satisfactorily, and consistently so, with HE.

3. *Taylor's blue.* This stain was developed in this laboratory (Taylor and Jeffree, 1969) and is routinely used with histological sections for the demonstration of metachromasia in cartilage matrix and connective tissue mucins. Its use in smears serves a similar purpose, for chondroid and mucinous intercellular matrix—when present in the tissue sampled—is always spread to some degree on the smeared

slide. It is thus of value in the identification of all chondroid smears, but particularly in the differentiation of giant-cell-containing chondroid lesions such as chondroblastoma and chondromyxoid fibroma from giant-cell tumour. Toluidine blue can be used as an alternative to Taylor's blue.

4 and 5. *PAS and PAS-diastase*. Two smears are stained with Periodic Acid Schiff (PAS), one of them after treatment with diastase. The technique helps in the identification of glycogen, neutral mucins and glycoproteins which are all PAS positive. Glycogen can be identified by its removal upon digestion with diastase; mucins and glycoproteins are diastase-resistant. Thus, PAS techniques are useful in the recognition of mucus-producing tumours and of tumours containing glycogen; the latter include cartilage tumours, Ewing's tumour and renal clear-cell carcinoma.

6. *Oil Red O*. This is used routinely on smears in this laboratory. There is a tendency to use fat stains only when a liposarcoma is suspected, but it is important for the cytodiagnostician and the histopathologist to appreciate that lipid material may accumulate in tumour cells of all sorts as a result of degenerative change, and to familiarize himself with the phenomenon. Oil Red O also helps demonstrate foam-cells in such conditions as Histiocytosis X, non-ossifying fibroma, giant-cell tumour and fibrous dysplasia.

7. *Alkaline phosphatase*. A preparation for the demonstration of alkaline phosphatase is indispensable and invaluable in bone tumour work. The enzyme is always present in osteosarcoma cells, whether these are of osteoblastic, chondroblastic, fibroblastic or anaplastic type. This enzyme is also present in endothelial cells and to some degree in adipose cells. Variable amounts of alkaline phosphatase may be present in some metastatic carcinomas.

8. *Acid phosphatase*. A preparation for the demonstration of acid phosphatase is another essential in bone tumour work. The enzyme is present in osteoclasts and histiocytes as well as in the cells of metastatic prostatic carcinoma. The acid phosphatase in prostatic carcinoma is formaldehyde-resistant and tartrate-inhibited, unlike that in osteoclasts and histiocytes. Relatively slight staining for acid phosphatase may be found in many other cells and this fact must be taken into account in cytochemical work.

9. *Beta-glucuronidase*. A preparation for the demonstration of this enzyme has been routinely used in this laboratory, mainly because it is richly present in plasma-cells, and in various lymphomas and leukaemias it may have a particular intra-cytoplasmic distribution (Jeffree, 1974).

In practice, however, it is of relatively minor practical value. The enzyme is practically ubiquitous and can be found in almost any cell. Furthermore, plasma-cell myeloma, lymphomas and leukaemias are more readily identifiable by routine staining procedures and one rarely relies on the demonstration of beta-glucuronidase for their diagnosis.

A number of other staining techniques are available for occasional use in selected cases, as and when required. They include:

10. *Perl's*. For the demonstration of haemosiderin. Haemosiderin is often found in non-ossifying fibroma, giant-cell tumour and reparative giant-cell granuloma.

11. *Neutral phosphatase.* A preparation for neutral phosphatase may have to be employed, with suitable control, when equivocal or paradoxical staining is observed with alkaline phosphatase preparations. Our technique for the demonstration of alkaline phosphatase may also demonstrate neutral phosphatase which is present in osteoclasts and these may then appear to be alkaline phosphatase positive. In such cases neutral phosphatase preparations will help establish the true nature of the enzyme.

12. *Mono-amine oxidase.* This is used with 'malignant round-cell tumours'. The enzyme is present in neuroblastoma cells whereas it is absent from the tumour cells in reticulosarcoma and Ewing's tumour.

13. *Masson–Fontana or Schmorl.* Either of these can be used, before and after bleaching, for the identification of melanin pigment. In bone tumour work the occasions for their use are, however, negligible.

14. *DOPA-oxidase.* A preparation for the demonstration of this enzyme will help in the diagnosis of metastatic amelanotic malignant melanoma, if the need rarely arises.

The technical details of the various routine stains and cytochemical procedures are set out in the Appendix to this volume (page 159).

References
Akerman M., Berg N.O. and Persson B.M. (1976) Fine needle aspiration biopsy in the evaluation of tumor-like lesions of bone. *Acta Orthop. Scand.* 47, 129.
Berg J.W. (1961) The aspiration biopsy smear. In: Koss L.G. (ed.), *Diagnostic Cytology and its Histopathologic Bases*. Philadelphia, Lippincott, p. 311.
Burstone M.S. (1958a) Histochemical comparison of Naphthol AS-Phosphates for the demonstration of phosphatases. *J. Natl. Cancer Inst.* 20, 601.
Burstone M.S. (1958b) Histochemical demonstration of acid phosphatases with Naphthol AS-Phosphates. *J. Natl. Cancer Inst.* 21, 523.
Burstone M.S. (1959) Histochemical demonstration of acid phospatase activity in osteoclasts. *J. Histochem. Cytochem.* 7, 39.
Cardozo P.L. (1954) *Clinical Cytology.* Leyden, Stasleu.
Cardozo P.L. (1975) *Atlas of Clinical Cytology.* Taiga b.v.'s-Herfogenbosch, Leiden, The Netherlands.
Changus G.W. (1957) Osteoblastic hyperplasia of bone: a histochemical appraisal of fibrous dysplasia of bone. *Cancer 10*, 1157.
Coley B.L., Sharp G.S. and Ellis E.B. (1931) Diagnosis of bone tumors by aspiration. *Am. J. Surg. 13*, 215.
Dudgeon L.S. and Barrett N.R. (1934) The examination of fresh tissues by the wet-film method. *Br. J. Surg. 22*, 4.
Dudgeon L.S. and Patrick C.V. (1927) A new method for the rapid microscopical diagnosis of tumours. *Br. J. Surg. 15*, 250.
Fell H.B. and Danielli J.F. (1943) The enzymes of healing wounds. I The distribution of alkaline phosphomonoesterase in experimental wounds and burns in the rat. *Br. J. Exp. Pathol. 24*, 196.
Fishman W.H. (1964) Rat skeletal muscle beta-glucuronidase localisation by post-coupling technique using Naphthol AS-BI-beta-D-glucosiduronic acid and Fast Dark Blue R. *J. Histochem. Cytochem. 12*, 306.
Fishman W.H. and Anlyan A.J. (1947) The presence of high beta-glucuronidase activity in cancer tissue. *J. Biol. Chem. 169*, 449.
Gomori G. (1939) Microtechnical demonstration of phosphatase in tissue sections. *Proc. Soc. Exp. Biol. Med. 42*, 23.
Gomori G. (1946) The study of enzymes in tissue sections. *Am. J. Clin. Pathol. 16*, 347.

Greep R.O., Fischer C.J. and Morse A. (1948) Alkaline phosphatase in odontogenesis and osteogenesis and its histochemical demonstration after demineralisation. *J. Am. Dent. Assoc. 36*, 427.

Hajdu S.I. and Hajdu E.O. (1976) *Cytopathology of Sarcomas and Other Nonepithelial Malignant Tumors.* Philadelphia, Saunders.

Hajdu S.I. and Melamed M.R. (1971) Needle biopsy of primary malignant bone tumors. *Surg. Gynecol. Obstet. 133*, 829.

Hayashi M., Nakajima Y. and Fishman W.H. (1964) The cytologic demonstration of beta-glucuronidase employing Naphthol AS-BI glucuronide and Hexazonium pararosanilin: a preliminary report. *J. Histochem. Cytochem. 12*, 293.

Jeffree G.M. (1969) Demonstration of beta-glucuronidase with Naphthol AS-BI-beta-D-glucosiduronic acid by simultaneous coupling. *J. Microsc. (Oxf.) 89*, 55.

Jeffree G.M. (1972) Enzymes in fibroblastic lesions: a histochemical and quantitative survey of alkaline and acid phosphatase, beta-glucuronidase, non-specific esterase and leucine aminopeptidase in benign and malignant fibroblastic lesions of bone and soft tissue. *J. Bone Joint Surg. 54-B*, 535.

Jeffree G.M. (1974) Enzymes of round cell tumours in bone and soft tissue: a histochemical survey. *J. Pathol. 113*, 101.

Jeffree G.M. and Price C.H.G. (1965) Bone tumours and their enzymes: a study of the phosphatases, non-specific esterases and beta-glucuronidase of osteogenic and cartilaginous tumours, fibroblastic and giant-cell lesions. *J. Bone Joint Surg. 47-B*, 120.

Kabat E.A. and Furth J. (1941) A histochemical study of the distribution of alkaline phosphatase in various normal and neoplastic tissues. *Am. J. Pathol. 17*, 303.

Manheimer L.H. and Seligman A.M. (1949) Improvement in method for histochemical demonstration of alkaline phosphatase and its use in the study of normal and neoplastic tissues. *J. Natl. Cancer Inst. 9*, 181.

Martin H.E. and Ellis E.B. (1930) Biopsy by needle puncture and aspiration. *Ann. Surg. 92*, 169.

Menten M.L., Junge J. and Green M.H. (1944) A coupling histochemical azo dye test for alkaline phosphatase in the kidney. *J. Biol. Chem. 153*, 471.

Monis B. and Rutenburg A.M. (1960) Alkaline phosphatase activity in neoplastic and inflammatory tissues of man. *Cancer 13*, 538.

Pepler W.J. (1958) The histochemistry of giant-cell tumours (osteoclastoma and giant-cell epulis). *J. Pathol. Bact. 76*, 505.

Robison R. (1923) The possible significance of hexosephosphoric esters in ossification. *Biochem. J. 17*, 286.

Robison R. and Soames K.M. (1924) The possible significance of hexosephosphoric esters in ossification. Part II, The phosphoric esterase of ossifying cartilage. *Biochem. J. 18*, 740.

Romanul F.C.A. and Bannister R.G. (1962) Localised areas of high alkaline phosphatase activity in the terminal arterial tree. *J. Cell Biol. 15*, 73.

Salzer-Kuntschik M. (1976) Cytologic and cytochemical behaviour of primary malignant bone tumors. In: Grundmann E. (ed.), *Malignant Bone Tumors*. Berlin, Springer-Verlag.

Schajowicz F. (1955) Aspiration biopsy in bone lesions: cytological and histological techniques. *J. Bone Joint Surg. 37-A*, 465.

Schajowicz F. (1961) Giant-cell tumors of bone (osteoclastoma): a pathological and histochemical study. *J. Bone Joint Surg. 43-A*, 1.

Schajowicz F. and Cabrini R.L. (1954) Histochemical studies of bone in normal and pathological conditions, with special reference to alkaline phosphatase, glycogen and mucopolysaccharides. *J. Bone Joint Surg. 36-B*, 474.

Schajowicz F. and Cabrini R.L. (1958) Histochemical localisation of acid phosphatase in bone tissue. *Science 127*, 1447.

Schajowicz F. and Derqui J.C. (1968) Puncture biopsy in lesions of the locomotor system: review of results in 4050 cases including 941 vertebral punctures. *Cancer 21*, 531.

Schajowicz F. and Hokama J. (1976) Aspiration (puncture or needle) biopsy in bone lesions. In: Grundmann E. (ed.), *Malignant Bone Tumors*. Berlin, Springer-Verlag.

Seligman A.M., Heymann H. and Barrnett R.J. (1954) The histochemical demonstration of alkaline phosphatase activity with indoxyl phosphate. *J. Histochem. Cytochem. 2*, 441.

Snyder R.E. and Coley B.L. (1945) Further studies on the diagnosis of bone tumors by aspiration biopsy. *Surg. Gynecol. Obstet. 80*, 517.

Söderström N. (1966) *Fine-needle Aspiration Biopsy: Used as a Direct Adjunct in Clinical Diagnostic Work.* Stockholm, Almqvist & Wicksell.

Stewart F.W. (1933) The diagnosis of tumors by aspiration. *Am. J. Pathol. 9*, 801.

Stormby N. and Akerman M. (1973) Cytodiagnosis of bone lesions by means of fine-needle aspiration biopsy. *Acta Cytol. 17*, 166.

Takamatsu H. (1939) Histologische und biochemische Studien über die Phosphatase (I. Mitteilung). Histochemische Untersuchungsmethodik der Phosphatase und deren Verteilung in verschiedenen Organen und Geweben. *Trans. Soc. Pathol. Japan* **29**, 492.

Taylor K.B. and Jeffree G.M. (1969) A new basic metachromatic dye, 1:9-Dimethyl Methylene Blue. *Histochem. J.* **1**, 199.

Thommesen P. and Frederiksen P. (1976) Fine needle aspiration biopsy of bone lesions: clinical value. *Acta Orthop. Scand.* **47**, 137.

Zajicek J. (1965) Sampling of cells from human tumours by aspiration biopsy for diagnosis and research. *Eur. J. Cancer.* **1**, 253.

Zajicek J. (1974) *Aspiration Biopsy Cytology*. Basel, Karger.

Chapter 2

Osteoblastic Lesions

Osteoblastic proliferation may occur in a variety of reactive processes, including fracture callus, periosteal reactions and myositis ossificans, in osteoid osteoma and osteoblastoma, and in osteosarcomas of various types.

In reactive proliferations, the constituent osteoblasts retain all the cytological features expected from normal osteoblasts, within the range of variation inherent in their development and maturation. In osteoid osteoma and osteoblastoma there is a variable, if relatively small, departure from the normal morphology. In osteosarcoma, the cell morphology always departs significantly from the normal, although in osteoblastic osteosarcomas the tumour cells can still be recognized as osteoblasts. In other types of osteosarcoma morphologically recognizable osteoblasts may be scanty or absent, so that the tumour cells can be recognized as of osteoblastic origin only by their cytochemical characteristics; they are all strongly alkaline phosphatase positive.

Thus, cytochemical demonstration of alkaline phosphatase is of great importance in the identification of osteoblasts and their precursors and neoplastic deviants. It should be mentioned here that osteoblasts are not the only connective tissue cells that are alkaline phosphatase positive, the exceptions being endothelial cells, adipocytes and 'hypertrophic' calcifying growth cartilage. Malignant endothelial cells and lipoblasts, like their normal cells of origin, may also contain alkaline phosphatase. Lipoblastic cells can be differentiated from osteosarcoma cells by their lipid content. Malignant endothelial cells cannot be cytochemically differentiated from anaplastic osteosarcoma cells and the diagnosis of angiosarcoma of bone will depend on its histological features; however, the latter is an extremely rare tumour, and this problem has never arisen in our experience. Chondrosarcoma, like growth cartilage, may in parts contain some alkaline phosphatase, but its enzyme content is variable and usually of low intensity. About half of all chondrosarcomas contain little or no alkaline phosphatase; nearly 40 % show alkaline phosphatase in only a fifth or less of the tumour cells; the remaining 10 % contain this enzyme in up to half of the tumour cells, mostly in relatively small amounts. In any case, the great majority of chondrosarcomas (*see* Chapter 3) can be readily differentiated from chondroblastic osteosarcoma on morphological criteria. In our experience the possible presence of alkaline phosphatase in these various non-osteoblastic cell types has not given rise to any great difficulty in practical diagnostic bone tumour work.

REACTIVE OSTEOBLASTIC PROLIFERATIONS
Fracture callus
Fracture callus and periosteal reactions are not usually biopsied unless they are

complications of some pathological process and are incidentally included in the excised tissue when biopsy is undertaken to determine the nature of the primary pathological lesion. Reactive new bone may often be included in biopsy material from various bone lesions, with or without pathological fracture, but in smears reactive osteoblasts derived therefrom are seen sparsely admixed with the predominant cells of the particular lesion biopsied. The significance and nature of such incidental reactive osteoblasts can be readily appreciated in the assessment of the preponderant lesional cells or cell varieties which they accompany.

The cytological characteristics of reactive osteoblasts derived from fracture callus (*Figs.* 2.1 and 2.2) are identical with those from myositis ossificans, which will be described in detail below.

Myositis ossificans

Myositis ossificans often presents as a rapidly developing mass in a muscle, with radiological evidence of increasing calcification over a short period of time, usually a matter of weeks. The clinical progression and radiological features should be characteristic enough to forewarn the surgeon against any surgical intervention. Nevertheless, for a variety of reasons—mostly from an anxiety not to miss a possible malignant growth such as soft-tissue osteosarcoma—the surgeon may have recourse to biopsy or excise these lesions. The general pathologist who rarely sees such lesions may, in his turn, view these florid proliferations with alarm and there is always the danger that they may be misdiagnosed as soft-tissue osteosarcomas. Indeed, this has been known to happen in our experience in the hands of the most competent of general histopathologists. It is not surprising, therefore, that the lesion has sometimes been called 'pseudomalignant osseous tumour of soft tissues' (Jaffe, 1958). For precisely the same reasons, florid subperiosteal reactive new bone has occasionally been mistaken by the uninitiated for osteosarcoma.

In myositis ossificans (*Figs.* 2.3–5), the lesional area has suffered extensive dissolution and disintegration of muscular tissue, providing a rich pabulum in which mesenchymal cells proliferate wildly as immature stellate or fibroblastic cells which actively undergo metaplasia into osteoblasts (*Figs.* 2.3–5). Frequent normal ...oses are present (*Fig.* 2.3). Remnants of damaged skeletal muscle, usually ...tly shrunken and disrupted and often represented by a mass of conglomerated ...lemmal nuclei (*Fig.* 2.4), may be found in the lesional area. The developing ...lasts organize themselves in a normal evolutionary manner and produce, ...sively, perfectly normal new bone (*Fig.* 2.5). By and large, this organiza- ...osteoid and eventually into mature bone is maximal and most advanced at ...ery from which the damaged area has been vascularized. This is in sharp ...ossifying osteosarcomas in which the peripheral or advancing zones of ...the least ossified.

...m myositis ossificans, in the early formative stages, show an ...steoblasts and fibroblasts (*Figs.* 2.6–10) and their less differentiated ...recursors which are seen as stellate or finely vacuolated round cells. ...can be readily found (*Fig.* 2.8) and are invariably of normal ...e osteoblasts present the usual variations in shape, some being ...ng, racket-shaped or sometimes of rectangular or truncated ...ere is only minimal variation in cytoplasmic and nuclear size, ...ccur only very occasionally (*Fig.* 2.6). The usual cytoplasmic ...cells, usually alongside the nucleus or at some slight distance ...learly in Giemsa stains (*Fig.* 2.7) and may be indistinct with

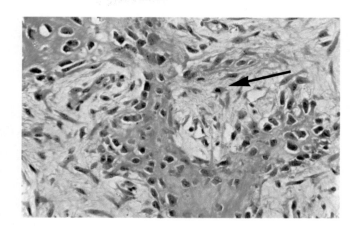

Fig. 2.1. **Fracture callus.** Reactive osteoblasts laying down osteoid. Adjoining tissue contains scattered fibroblasts, one of which is in mitosis (arrowed). Compare with myositis ossificans (*Fig.* 2.5) at a similar stage of development. (HE × 192.)

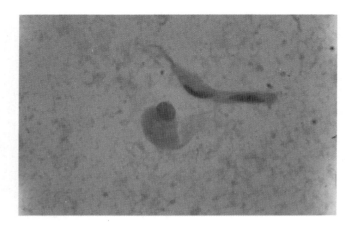

Fig. 2.2. **Fracture callus.** Smear showing typical osteoblast. The two fusiform cells above are almost certainly endothelial cells. In alkaline phosphatase preparations the endothelial cells as well as the osteoblasts would stain positively. (HE × 480.)

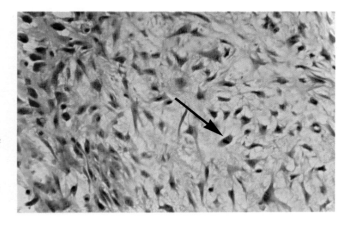

Fig. 2.3. **Myositis ossificans.** Histology shows florid proliferation of stellate and fusiform mesenchymal cells, with early differentiation into osteoblasts at the left margin of the field. Mitosis arrowed. (HE × 192.)

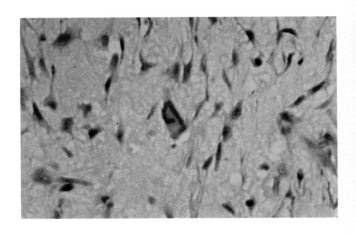

Fig. 2.4. **Myositis ossificans.** Same case as in Fig. 2.3. Shrunken damaged muscle fibre is seen at the centre of the field. Sarcolemmal nuclei have agglomerated, so that the structure appears as a 'multinucleate giant cell'. (HE × 307.)

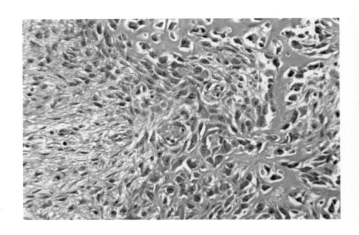

Fig. 2.5. **Myositis ossificans.** Another case. Fibroblastic proliferation (on the left), undergoing metaplasia into osteoblasts (central zone), with deposition of osteoidal matrix (on right). Compare with fracture callus (*Fig. 2.1*). (HE × 192.)

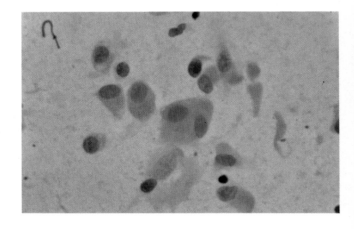

Fig. 2.6. **Myositis ossificans.** Same case as in Fig. 2.5. Smear showing reactive osteoblasts, including a binucleate cell. Compare with osteoid osteoma (*Fig. 2.13*), osteoblastoma (*Fig. 2.16*) and well-differentiated osteoblastic osteosarcoma (*Fig. 2.22*). (HE × 480.)

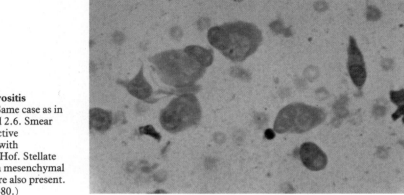

Fig. 2.7. **Myositis ossificans.** Same case as in *Figs.* 2.5 and 2.6. Smear showing reactive osteoblasts, with cytoplasmic Hof. Stellate and fusiform mesenchymal precursors are also present. (Giemsa × 480.)

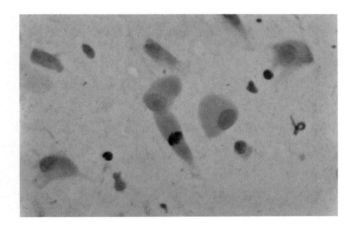

Fig. 2.8. **Myositis ossificans.** Same case as in *Figs.* 2.3 and 2.4. Smear showing reactive osteoblasts and fusiform precursors, one of them in mitosis. (HE × 480.)

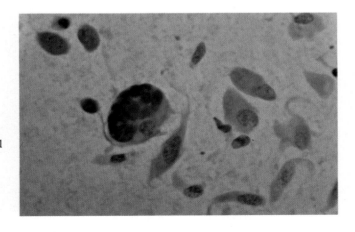

Fig. 2.9. **Myositis ossificans.** Same case as in *Figs.* 2.5–7. Smear showing reactive osteoblasts and spindle cells. Also shrunken remnant of damaged skeletal muscle fibre, with agglomeration of its sarcolemmal nuclei. Compare with osteoclast shown in *Fig.* 2.14. (HE × 480.)

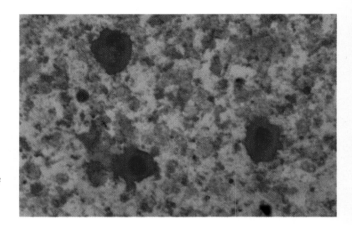

Fig. 2.10. **Myositis ossificans.** Same case as in *Figs.* 2.5–7 and 2.9. Smear: reactive osteoblasts staining strongly positive for alkaline phosphatase. (Alkaline phosphatase preparation × 480.)

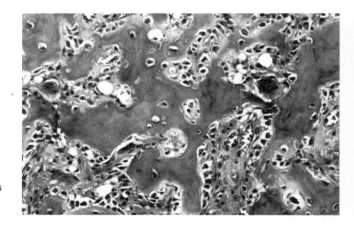

Fig. 2.11. **Osteoid osteoma.** Histology shows osteoblastic proliferation with production of osteoid and new bone. Note presence of scattered osteoclasts which are always present in developing bone. (HE × 192.)

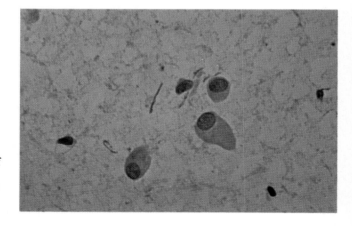

Fig. 2.12. **Osteoid osteoma.** Smear showing representative osteoblasts. Compare with osteoblasts of myositis ossificans (*Fig.* 2.6–9) and of osteoblastoma (*Figs.* 2.16–18). (HE × 480.)

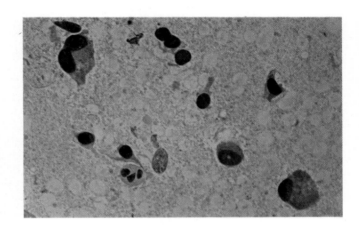

Fig. 2.13. **Osteoid osteoma.** Smear showing scattered osteoblasts, including a binucleate cell. Compare nuclear size in binucleate cells of myositis ossificans (*Fig.* 2.6), osteoblastoma (*Fig.* 2.16) and well-differentiated osteoblastic osteosarcoma (*Fig.* 2.22). (HE × 480.)

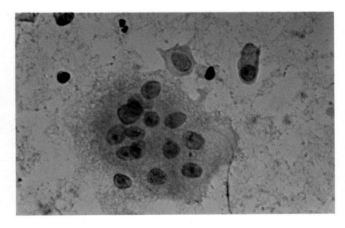

Fig. 2.14. **Osteoid osteoma.** Smear showing a typical osteoclast and several osteoblasts. Nuclei of osteoblasts are roughly the same size as the nuclei of the osteoclast. Osteoclasts can be found in most smears from various bone lesions, and their nuclei provide a good guide to the assessment of nuclear size in other cells. (HE × 480.)

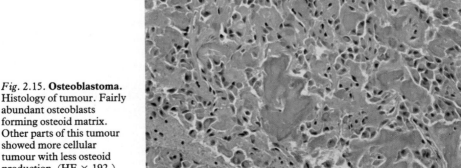

Fig. 2.15. **Osteoblastoma.** Histology of tumour. Fairly abundant osteoblasts forming osteoid matrix. Other parts of this tumour showed more cellular tumour with less osteoid production. (HE × 192.)

HE. The nucleus normally lies at or very near the cell membrane at one pole, and may sometimes appear as though it is being extruded from the cell (*Fig.* 2.7). Remnants of damaged muscle (*Fig.* 2.9) may also be seen in smears, appearing as multinucleate giant cells because of the approximation of the sarcolemmal nuclei following shrinkage or disappearance of the sarcoplasm; they should not be mistaken for multinucleate histiocytes, tumour giant-cells or osteoclasts. Osteoclasts are present in variable numbers, for they are always to be found in developing bone and in smears prepared therefrom.

The osteoblasts, and to a lesser degree their stellate and fusiform precursors, contain alkaline phosphatase in their cytoplasm (*Fig.* 2.10). In the preparation of smears a fair proportion of the cells always rupture, discharging their enzyme-rich contents. For this reason, the background of osteoblast-rich smears stains positively, and to the naked eye such slides appear distinctly brick-red in colour.

OSTEOID OSTEOMA
The lesional tissue of osteoid osteoma (*Fig.* 2.11) is said to bear a close resemblance to benign osteoblastoma and some authors believe that it may be indistinguishable from the latter except by its smaller size (Byers, 1968; Schajowicz and Lemos, 1970), the maximal diameter for osteoid osteoma being variously taken as 1 cm or 2 cm. Although there is no consensus of opinion as to the precise nature of osteoid osteoma, many consider it to be a benign neoplastic lesion allied to osteoblastoma (Schajowicz and Lemos, 1970; Spjut et al., 1971; Lichtenstein, 1972). Its clinical and radiological features are quite distinct from those of osteoblastoma (Pochaczevsky et al., 1960; Lichtenstein, 1956, 1972) and usually render its firm diagnosis possible before excision. It is often excised *en bloc* with the surrounding sclerotic host bone and smears from it are seldom made. The only example in our records with available smears was unusual because of its large size (3 cm diam.) and was clinically suspected to be an inflammatory lesion. In view of its size, most would consider it as an example of osteoblastoma, but Lichtenstein (1972) would regard it as a giant-sized osteoid osteoma.

Smears easily and promptly proved it to be a benign osteoblastic lesion, not an inflammatory one. Since osteoidal and bony matrix forms a substantial part of the lesion, the cell population derived from its smears is sparse, essentially osteoblasts (*Figs.* 2.12–14) with a sprinkling of fibrocytes and osteoclasts (*Fig.* 2.14). The osteoblasts show none of the features expected in osteosarcoma. Mitoses are absent, but occasional binucleate osteoblasts can be seen (*Fig.* 2.13). Alkaline phosphatase is demonstrable, as expected, in the lesional cells.

OSTEOBLASTOMA
Osteoblastoma is a rare neoplastic proliferation of osteoblasts with production of osteoidal matrix. Since its first recognition and designation as 'giant osteoid osteoma' (Dahlin and Johnson, 1954), its histological resemblance to osteoid osteoma has been stressed. Despite this, most examples are histologically distinguishable from osteoid osteoma (Lichtenstein, 1956, 1972) and, indeed, some cases may present formidable difficulty in their histological differentation from osteosarcoma. A malignant or aggressive variant of osteoblastoma has now been recognized (Mayer, 1967; Schajowicz and Lemos, 1976).

Only 9 examples of osteoblastoma have been recorded in the 32-year history of this Registry, compared with 45 examples of osteoid osteoma, and only a few cases have come to be smeared for cytological examination.

One example was a rather cellular osteoblastoma (*Fig.* 2.15) of the talus, which recurred and necessitated amputation of the foot; it was indeed considered by a panel of bone tumour pathologists as a 'malignant' osteoblastoma. Its smears show an abundance of recognizable osteoblasts (*Figs.* 2.16–19) among which binucleate cells are relatively frequent (*Figs.* 2.16 and 2.18); the latter can be found practically in every medium-sized microscopic field. The lesional cells contain alkaline phosphatase (*Fig.* 2.19). Occasional mitoses can be found (*Fig.* 2.17). The cell morphology, particularly in regard to nuclear size and appearance, is quite different from that seen in a well-differentiated osteosarcoma; it is also noticeably different from that of reactive osteoblastic proliferations. A comparison of the nuclear size in binucleate cells is given below in black-and-white tracings, drawn at the same magnification, from myositis ossificans, osteoid osteoma, osteoblastoma and osteosarcoma.

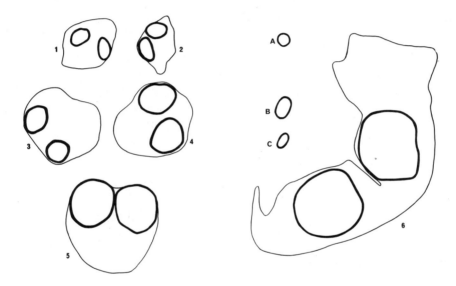

Line drawings of binucleate cells from myositis ossificans, osteoid osteoma, osteoblastoma and osteosarcoma. Osteoclast and small lymphocyte nuclei have also been drawn for comparison.
These and all line drawings in subsequent chapters have been drawn at the same magnification.
1. Myositis ossificans (cell from *Fig.* 2.6).
2. Osteoid osteoma (cell from *Fig.* 2.13).
3. Osteoblastoma (cell from *Fig.* 2.16).
4. Osteoblastic osteosarcoma (cell from *Fig.* 2.29).
5. Osteoblastic osteosarcoma (cell from *Fig.* 2.22).
6. Anaplastic (telangiectatic) osteosarcoma (cell from *Fig.* 2.52).
A. Nucleus of small lymphocyte (from a tuberculous smear, *Fig.* 8.8, Chapter 8). The nuclei of small lymphocytes seen in the smear of a lymphoblastic lymphosarcoma (*Fig.* 6.2, Chapter 6) are also of similar size.
B. Nucleus of juvenile osteoclast (*Fig.* 2.14). Nuclei of juvenile osteoclasts are larger than those of mature osteoclasts.
C. Nucleus of mature osteoclast (*Fig.* 5.18, Chapter 5).
Outline drawings show the nuclear size in myositis ossificans and osteoid osteoma to be similar. Nuclei in osteosarcoma are demonstrably, and at times dramatically, larger. Nuclear size in osteoblastoma occupies an intermediate position.

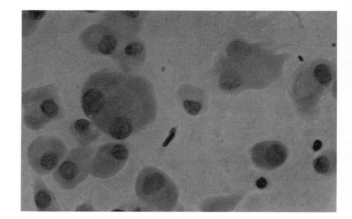

Fig. 2.16. **Osteoblastoma.**
Osteoblast-rich smear.
Compare with cells of
myositis ossificans (*Fig.*
2.6), osteoid osteoma (*Fig.*
2.13) and osteoblastic
osteosarcoma (*Figs.* 2.21,
2.22, 2.24, 2.25, 2.28,
2.29). (HE × 480.)

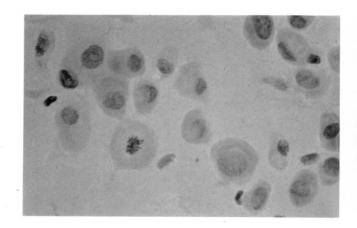

Fig. 2.17. **Osteoblastoma.**
Smear showing
representative osteoblasts,
including a large cell with
large open nucleus and one
in mitosis. (HE × 480.)

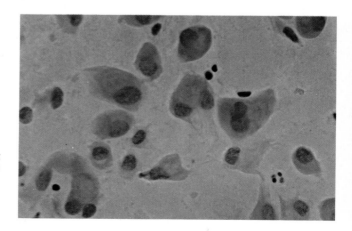

Fig. 2.18. **Osteoblastoma.**
Field from smear containing
three binucleate osteoblasts;
the latter are relatively rare
in reactive osteoblastic
proliferations and in osteoid
osteoma. (HE × 480.)

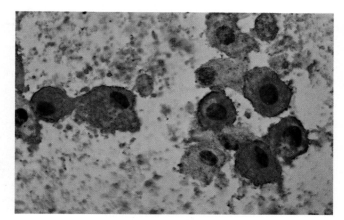

Fig. 2.19. **Osteoblastoma.**
Smear: tumour cells staining
positively for alkaline
phosphatase. (Alkaline
phosphatase
preparation × 480.)

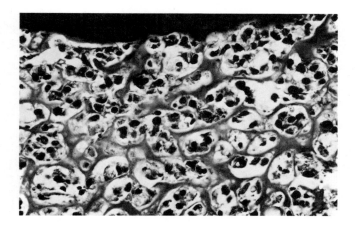

Fig. 2.20. **Osteoblastic
osteosarcoma.** Case 1.
Histology of tumour,
showing abundant osteoid
matrix. (HE × 192.)

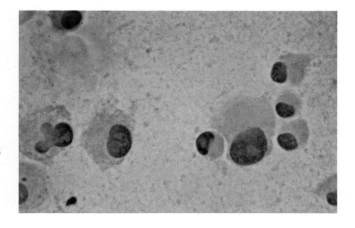

Fig. 2.21. **Osteoblastic
osteosarcoma.** Case 1.
Smear: morphologically
recognizable osteoblasts
with variation in size of cells
and nuclei. Nuclear
chromatin dark; large
nucleoli. Abnormal
lobulation of nucleus
(extreme left). (HE × 480.)

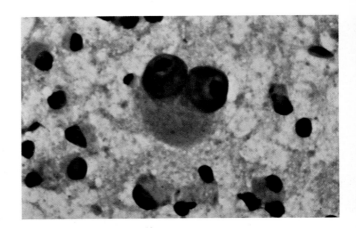

Fig. 2.22. **Osteoblastic osteosarcoma.** Case 1. Smear showing giant binucleate malignant osteoblast with huge nucleoli. Compare with binucleate osteoblasts of myositis ossificans (*Fig.* 2.6), osteoid osteoma (*Fig.* 2.13) and osteoblastoma (*Fig.* 2.16). (Giemsa × 480.)

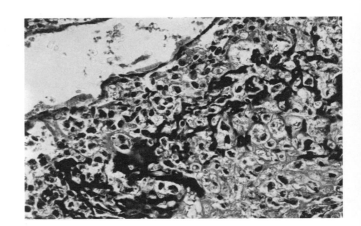

Fig. 2.23. **Osteoblastic osteosarcoma.** Case 2. Typical deposition of tumour osteoid. (HE × 192.)

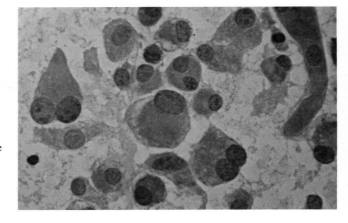

Fig. 2.24. **Osteoblastic osteosarcoma.** Case 2. Smear showing group of tumour cells with variations in cell and nuclear size. Nuclear chromatin more open than in *Case* 1. A large mononucleate cell with large nucleus and several binucleate cells are present. Compare with osteoblastoma (*Fig.* 2.16). (HE × 480.)

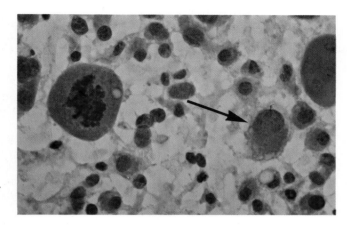

Fig. 2.25. **Osteoblastic osteosarcoma.** Case 2. Smear showing group of tumour cells, including a giant tumour cell in mitosis. Part of an osteoclast is shown (top right); compare size of its nuclei with nucleus of adjoining tumour osteoblast (arrowed). (HE × 480.)

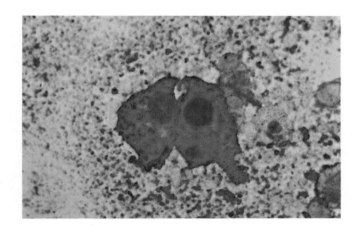

Fig. 2.26. **Osteoblastic osteosarcoma.** Case 2. Smear: tumour cells rich in alkaline phosphatase. (Alkaline phosphatase preparation × 480.)

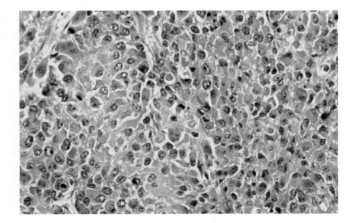

Fig. 2.27. **Osteoblastic osteosarcoma.** Case 3. Histologically moderately differentiated, with scanty tumour osteoid. (HE × 192.)

OSTEOSARCOMA

Osteosarcoma is defined in conventional histological terms as a malignant tumour of bone which shows evidence of osteoid production by the tumour cells. It may be predominantly osteoblastic, chondroblastic, fibroblastic or anaplastic; rare varieties include the telangiectatic and giant-celled forms. Mixed osteosarcomas occur in which the various patterns may be found in different parts of the tumour. A special variety, with much better prognosis and a characteristic histological pattern, is parosteal osteosarcoma; it will be separately and briefly discussed at the end of this chapter.

A firm diagnosis of osteosarcoma is not always possible on routine histological examination of limited, and sometimes even of extensive, samples of a malignant bone tumour, in that no tumour osteoid may be demonstrable. The sampled tumour tissue may be entirely spindle-celled or fibroblastic, chondroblastic or anaplastic, in which case a variety of other diagnoses may be arrived at, including fibrosarcoma in the case of spindle-celled sarcomas, chondrosarcoma when the tumour is exclusively chondroblastic, anaplastic sarcoma with undifferentiated growths or 'giant-cell sarcoma' with predominantly giant-celled tumours. When further material becomes available for histological examination, for instance after amputation, tumour osteoid may be found to prove the fundamentally osteosarcomatous nature of such tumours.

It has been our experience that a firm cytological diagnosis of osteosarcoma can confidently be made on cytomorphological and cytochemical criteria in all cases, however bizarre the histological picture and whether osteoid is present or not in the biopsied tumour.

On cell morphology alone only tumours showing some recognizable osteoblastic differentiation can be confidently diagnosed as osteosarcoma. A diagnosis of sarcoma can be readily made on smears of all the other variants of osteosarcoma, but indication of their osteoblastic derivation requires the demonstration of abundant alkaline phosphatase in their cytoplasm. A sarcomatous smear, easily recognizable as such in routine smears stained with HE, Giemsa or Taylor's blue, which is richly alkaline phosphatase positive is, to all practical intents and purposes, osteosarcoma.

All osteosarcoma cells, whatever the predominant histological pattern or cytological morphology in any given example, are richly alkaline phosphatase positive. Fibrosarcoma, which may be confused with fibroblastic osteosarcoma, is alkaline phosphatase negative. Chondrosarcoma, in the great majority of cases, is either alkaline phosphatase negative or contains variable, often relatively low, amounts of this enzyme in a small proportion of the tumour cells. About 10 % of chondrosarcomas, including the low-grade varieties, may show alkaline phosphatase activity in up to half of the tumour cells, but the great majority of these cases can be separated cytomorphologically from chondroblastic osteosarcoma. It is theoretically possible that an occasional high-grade chondrosarcoma with abundant alkaline phosphatase might occur, but we have not yet come across such a case. In that eventuality, the precise categorization of the tumour would depend on full assessment of all collateral information available, including the clinical and radiological features and a detailed histological examination.

Two other extremely rare intra-osseous sarcomas might conceivably give rise to a diagnostic problem, namely liposarcoma and angiosarcoma, the component cells of which might be expected to contain alkaline phosphatase. No example of liposarcoma or angiosarcoma of bone has been recorded in this Registry. In the case of liposarcoma, lipid should be demonstrable in a fair proportion of the tumour cells in both cytological smears and in cryostat sections. In the case of angiosarcoma, which should not be confused with telangiectatic osteosarcoma, as it sometimes is, subsequent histological sections should suffice to establish the correct diagnosis.

Osteoblastic osteosarcoma

Osteoblastic osteosarcoma is histologically characterized by a predominant proliferation of malignant osteoblasts laying down osteoidal matrix to a greater or lesser degree (*Figs*. 2.20, 2.23 and 2.27).

Smears from osteoblastic osteosarcomas (*Figs*. 2.21, 2.22, 2.24–26, 2.28 and 2.29) yield an abundance of cells which are manifestly identifiable as osteoblastic on morphological criteria. There is appreciable nuclear and cytoplasmic pleomorphism and numbers of exceptionally large cells with hyperchromatic giant or multiple nuclei can be found (*Fig*. 2.22). The nuclei are considerably larger, with more open coarsely stippled chromatin network or with darker diffuse chromatin, and larger nucleoli than in osteoblastoma. Mitoses (*Fig*. 2.25) are always present in fair numbers, in sharp contrast to osteoblastoma, and some of them are of abnormal type. All the tumour cells are stongly alkaline phosphatase positive (*Fig*. 2.26). The less differentiated variants of osteoblastic osteosarcoma (*Figs*. 2.30–32) increasingly lose their morphological osteoblastic characteristics and merge into the group of anaplastic osteosarcomas to be discussed later in this chapter.

It must be stressed that in well-differentiated osteoblastic osteosarcomas individual tumour cells or small groups of cells can be selected which, viewed in isolation and out of context of the smear as a whole, may be difficult to differentiate from those of reactive proliferations or of osteoblastoma. However, throughout the smear are frequent mononucleate tumour cells which may be twice or more the size of comparable cells in osteoblastoma, and their nuclei are also proportionately larger and more primitive (*Figs*. 2.22, 2.24). Huge binucleate or multinucleate cells can be found (*Fig*. 2.22). This malignant pleomorphism, coupled with the frequence of mitoses and the presence of abnormal mitoses, is the clearest cytological indication separating well-differentiated osteoblastic osteosarcoma from osteoblastoma, the only condition with which it could remotely be confused in cytological smears. The cytology of fracture callus and myositis ossificans, alias 'pseudosarcomatous osseous tumour of soft tissues', is singularly of benign or normal type, despite the frequency of mitoses, and it is difficult to see how they could be mistaken for osteosarcoma.

Chondroblastic osteosarcoma

In chondroblastic osteosarcoma (*Figs*. 2.33 and 2.39) the predominant proliferation is not by morphologically recognizable osteoblasts but by deviants of them, which have undergone some transformation or metaplasia into primitive cartilage cells. This transformation is not universal throughout the tumour, nor is it total in any given cell, so that the tumour cells retain some of the functional and enzymatic characteristics expected in untransformed malignant osteoblasts. Depending on their degree of differentiation and transformation, the tumour cells in chondroblas-

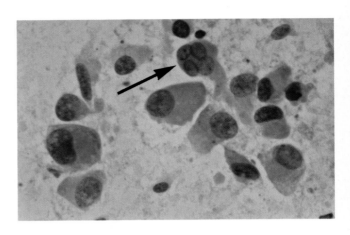

Fig. 2.28. **Osteoblastic osteosarcoma.** Case 3. Smear showing group of malignant osteoblasts, all with large dark nuclei; nuclear size several times greater than that of osteoclast (arrowed). (HE × 480.)

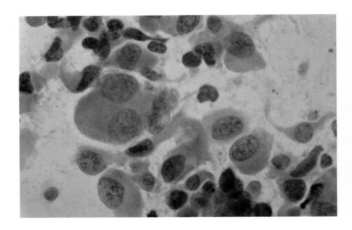

Fig. 2.29. **Osteoblastic osteosarcoma.** Case 3. Smear showing malignant pleomorphism of tumour osteoblasts. A binucleate cell is present. Nuclei are exceptionally large, compared with those of osteoblastoma (*Figs.* 2.16–18). (HE × 480.)

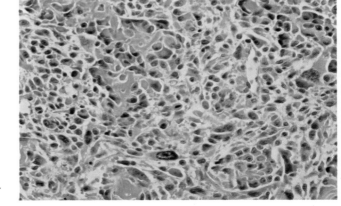

Fig. 2.30. **Osteoblastic osteosarcoma.** Case 4. Histologically somewhat poorly differentiated, with scattered tumour giant-cells. (HE × 192.)

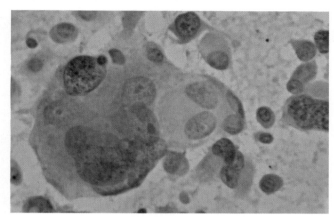

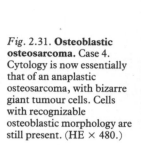

Fig. 2.31. **Osteoblastic osteosarcoma.** Case 4. Cytology is now essentially that of an anaplastic osteosarcoma, with bizarre giant tumour cells. Cells with recognizable osteoblastic morphology are still present. (HE × 480.)

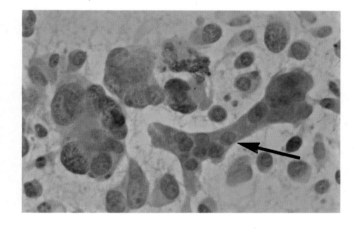

Fig. 2.32. **Osteoblastic osteosarcoma.** Case 4. Smear: some osteoblastic morphology is still identifiable in a proportion of the tumour cells; otherwise essentially an anaplastic osteosarcoma. Compare size of nuclei in giant tumour cells with those in osteoclast (arrowed). (HE × 480.)

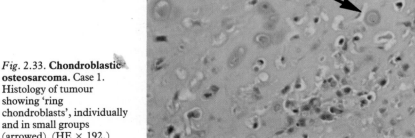

Fig. 2.33. **Chondroblastic osteosarcoma.** Case 1. Histology of tumour showing 'ring chondroblasts', individually and in small groups (arrowed). (HE × 192.)

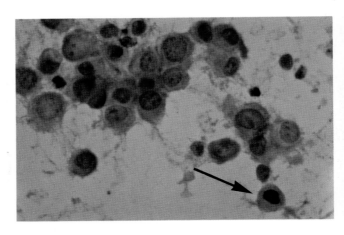

Fig. 2.34. **Chondroblastic osteosarcoma.** Case 1. Smear showing cluster of immature chondroblastic tumour cells. Large nuclei with relatively fine chromatin, one or two fine nucleoli, pale cytoplasm. Cell in mitosis (arrowed). A few specks of background metachromasia. (Taylor's blue × 480.)

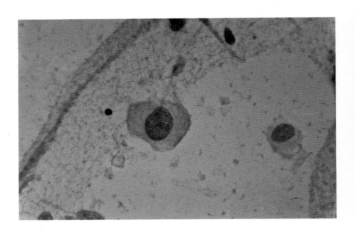

Fig. 2.35. **Chondroblastic osteosarcoma.** Case 1. Smear: two chondroblastic tumour cells, one much larger and more primitive than the other. Cytoplasm pale and very finely vacuolated. Background is lightly metachromatic due to presence of mucoid material. (Taylor's blue × 480.)

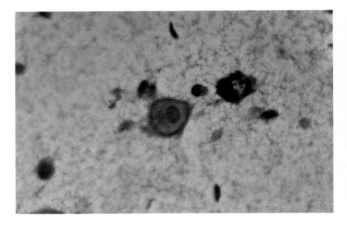

Fig. 2.36. **Chondroblastic osteosarcoma.** Case 1. Smear shows maturing chondroblast with a ring of metachromatic matrix surrounding it—a 'ring chondroblast' (note similar cells in histological section, *Fig.* 2.33). (Taylor's blue × 480.)

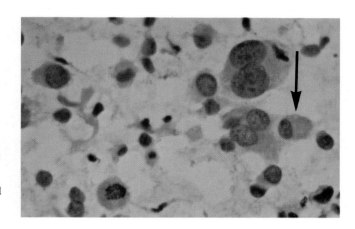

Fig. 2.37. **Chondroblastic osteosarcoma.** Case 1. Smear: group of tumour cells, including two binucleate cells, one much larger than the other. Some cells show tendency to osteoblastic differentiation (arrowed). Also tumour cell in mitosis (bottom left). (HE × 480.)

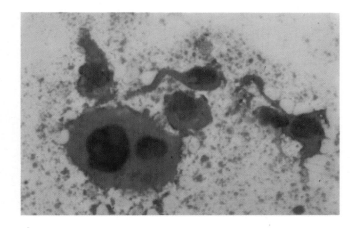

Fig. 2.38. **Chondroblastic osteosarcoma.** Case 1. Smear: tumour cells, including a giant form, richly alkaline phosphatase positive. (Alkaline phosphatase preparation × 480.)

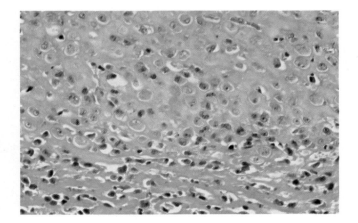

Fig. 2.39. **Chondroblastic osteosarcoma.** Case 2. Histology of tumour: chondroid above, osteoblastic below. (HE × 192.)

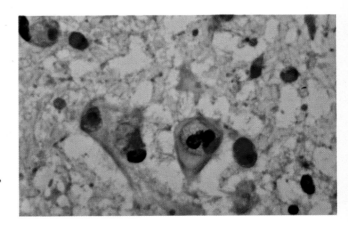

Fig. 2.40. **Chondroblastic osteosarcoma.** Case 2. Smear showing mature tumour chondroblast with atypical double nucleus. Nucleus is surrounded by a circular vacuolated zone, beyond which some eosinophilic material has been deposited. Other cells are in various stages of degeneration and shrinkage, and many have eosinophilic orange-red cytoplasm. (HE × 480.)

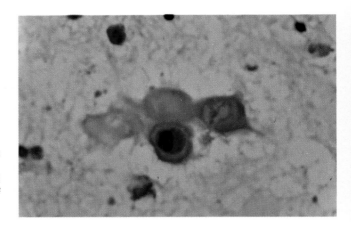

Fig. 2.41. **Chondroblastic osteosarcoma.** Case 2. Smear: typical developed 'ring chondroblast' with well-defined ring of dense orange-red matrix surrounding it. The nucleus appears dark and condensed. Three adjoining similar cells have undergone necrosis and are devoid of nuclei. (HE × 480.)

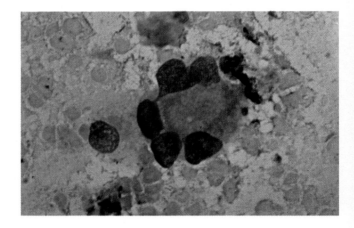

Fig. 2.42. **Chondroblastic osteosarcoma.** Case 2. Smear showing giant multinucleate tumour cell. (Giemsa × 480.)

Fig. 2.43. **Chondroblastic osteosarcoma.** Case 2. Smear showing group of typical chondroblastic tumour cells, including a characteristic 'ring chondroblast' and two undifferentiated cells. Compare the nuclear and cytoplasmic features of the immature and mature cells. The nucleus of the mature cell has condensed chromatin network and is smaller. The cytoplasm has metachromatic mucoid material in its substance; similar material has condensed in a ring around the cell. (Taylor's blue × 480.)

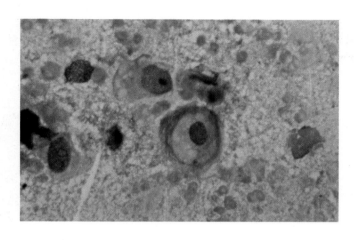

Fig. 2.44. **Chondroblastic osteosarcoma.** Case 2. Smear: tumour giant-cell in abnormal mitosis. Note that the magnification of this illustration is nearly half that of the other cytological pictures. (HE × 307.)

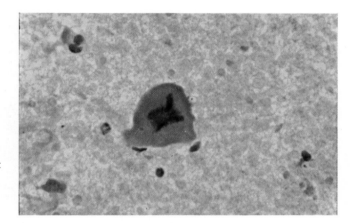

Fig. 2.45. **Fibroblastic osteosarcoma.** Histology of tumour: a spindle-cell sarcoma, without any osteoid matrix, which might be diagnosed as a fibrosarcoma in the absence of enzyme studies. (HE × 192.)

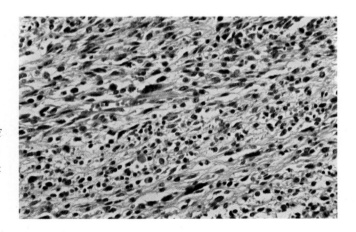

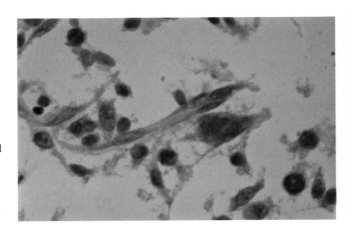

Fig. 2.46. **Fibroblastic osteosarcoma.** Smear showing an admixture of ovoid and fusiform tumour cells, including a multinucleate giant cell. Cell preservation is rather imperfect, because the amputation specimen was received from abroad many days after amputation. (HE × 480.)

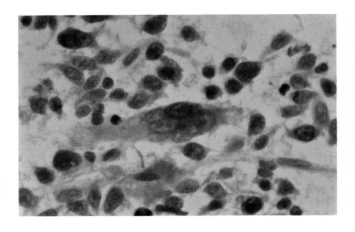

Fig. 2.47. **Fibroblastic osteosarcoma.** Smear showing typical fusiform tumour giant cell with multiple nucleolated nuclei. Also admixture of rounded, ovoid and fusiform tumour cells. (HE × 480.)

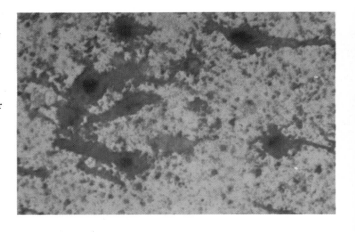

Fig. 2.48. **Fibroblastic osteosarcoma.** Smear showing tumour cells, many clearly fusiform and fibroblast-like, containing abundant alkaline phosphatase. Compare with fibrosarcoma cells (*Figs.* 4.10, 4.15 and 4.16, Chapter 4) which are devoid of alkaline phosphatase. Note that autolysis of several days' duration has not adversely affected the enzyme content of the tumour cells. (Alkaline phosphatase preparation × 480.)

tic osteosarcoma may lay down matrix which is chondroid or chondro-osteoid. A variable, but usually small, percentage of the tumour cells may remain essentially untransformed malignant osteoblasts and lay down osteoid matrix in parts of the tumour.

Smears from chondroblastic osteosarcoma may thus show a number of cells similar to the malignant osteoblasts of osteoblastic osteosarcoma. The predominant chondroblastic or chondro-osteoblastic cell (*Figs.* 2.34, 2.35 and 2.43) is round or ovoid, has a large round or ovoid nucleus with one or two usually fine nucleoli and delicate chromatin tending to condense at the nuclear margins. Cells with double and, sometimes, multiple nuclei are not infrequent (*Figs.* 2.37, 2.38, 2.40 and 2.42). Mitoses can easily be found (*Figs.* 2.34, 2.37 and 2.44) and may be abnormal (*Fig.* 2.44). The cytoplasm is generally pale and may be finely stippled or granular. With increasing maturity or differentiation, the cytoplasm progressively increases in volume, becomes coarsely or finely vacuolated, and eosinophilic material is deposited circumferentially along the cytoplasmic border (*Fig.* 2.40). In the most differentiated cells (*Figs.* 2.36, 2.40 and 2.41), the peripheral eosinophilic material broadens, becomes dense and hyaline, and encases the cell as an eosinophilic orange-red ring; it is metachromatic with Taylor's blue (*Figs.* 2.36 and 2.43) and is clearly chondroid matrix. Such 'ring chondroblasts' may be seen individually or in small clusters in histological sections from chondroblastic osteosarcoma (*Fig.* 2.33). With these cytoplasmic changes, there is a corresponding condensation and pyknosis of the nuclei, which become smaller, darker and often elongated. Numbers of degenerate or necrotic shrunken cells, staining orange-red with eosin, are scattered throughout the smear (*Fig.* 2.40) and necrotic unshrunken 'ring chondroblasts' (*Fig.* 2.41) can also be seen. Cells intermediate between chondroblastic and osteoblastic forms also occur (*Fig.* 2.37). Alkaline phosphatase is demonstrable in all types of tumour cells (*Fig.* 2.38) derived from chondroblastic osteosarcoma.

The cytomorphological and cytochemical differentiation of chondroblastic osteosarcoma from chondrosarcoma has already been outlined in the introduction to osteosarcomas (p. 19) and will be further discussed in the Chapter on cartilage tumours (p. 60).

Fibroblastic osteosarcoma

Fibroblastic osteosarcoma (*Fig.* 2.45) is a predominantly spindle-celled sarcoma which lays down fibrous matrix but also shows a limited amount of tumour osteoid; part of the matrix may be intermediate between the two, in the form of fibro-osteoid and may subsequently undergo ossification. Demonstration of tumour osteoid is essential for the histological diagnosis of fibroblastic osteosarcoma, otherwise it is impossible to distinguish it from fibrosarcoma in routine histological sections. Unfortunately, osteoid formation may be remarkably scanty in fibroblastic osteosarcoma and need not necessarily be sampled at biopsy. For this reason, a number of fibroblastic osteosarcomas are diagnosed as fibrosarcomas or spindle-cell sarcomas, unless cytochemistry or histochemistry has been performed. The tumour cells in fibroblastic osteosarcoma are all alkaline phosphatase positive (*Fig.* 2.48), whereas they are alkaline phosphatase negative in fibrosarcoma.

Depending on the degree of differentiation of a given tumour, smears from fibroblastic osteosarcoma show an admixture of round or ovoid primitive cells and spindle-shaped or fusiform cells (*Figs.* 2.46, 2.47). Both normal and abnormal mitoses are demonstrable. Tumour giant-cells are present and often have an elongated or fusiform configuration, although numbers of rounded or bizarre giant cells may also occur.

Telangiectatic osteosarcoma

Telangiectatic osteosarcoma is basically an anaplastic osteosarcoma (*Figs.* 2.49–51) whose stroma contains an abundant and extensive network of aneurysmal vascular spaces (*Fig.* 2.49), in its general architectural structure resembling an aneurysmal bone cyst, the delicate septa separating the aneurysmal channels being populated by the tumour cells (*Fig.* 2.50). The sarcoma cells are often bizarre and pleomorphic, abnormal mitoses and tumour giant-cells abound, and no identifiable endothelium separates the tumour tissue from the aneurysmal spaces. A variable sprinkling of osteoclasts, often tending to border the vascular lumen, can be found among the tumour cells. Tumour osteoid can normally be found in some part of the tumour (*Fig.* 2.51), but may require careful search for its discovery.

Smears from telangiectatic osteosarcoma are illustrated in *Figs.* 2.52–55. Morphologically they present the cytological features of a pleomorphic bizarre sarcoma. Cytochemically, abundant alkaline phosphatase is demonstrable in the tumour cells (*Fig.* 2.55).

Because of its architectural resemblance to aneurysmal bone cyst, telangiectatic osteosarcoma may occasionally be misdiagnosed for the former, but this confusion is totally unwarranted both on histological and cytological criteria. Another possible confusion is with angiosarcoma; indeed, some angiosarcomas so diagnosed are really examples of telangiectatic osteosarcoma. We suspect that a sharp differentiation of telangiectatic osteosarcoma from angiosarcoma might not be possible on purely cytological criteria, since both vascular endothelium and osteoblasts contain alkaline phosphatase. Angiosarcoma of bone is, however, a tumour of extreme rarity and the problem must remain a largely theoretical one.

Anaplastic osteosarcoma

In some osteosarcomas, the tumour may not be demonstrably osteoblastic, chondroblastic or fibroblastic, or some admixture of these, but may present a variety of pleomorphic or unusual histological patterns and only meticulous search may demonstrate tumour osteoid as part of their matrix. Whatever the cytological morphology of these tumours, their cells are shown to contain alkaline phosphatase.

Some cases may be histologically designated as 'giant-cell sarcomas', an unfortunate term since it gives rise to possible confusion with giant-cell tumours (osteoblastomas). The term 'giant-cell sarcoma' has at times been applied to two different types of osteosarcoma:

1. *Osteosarcoma in which there is an over-abundance of tumour giant cells*

The striking feature of these is the abundance of abnormal giant cells (*Figs.* 2.56–60) with highly polyploid nuclei which undergo bizarre or multipolar mitosis to produce large numbers of hyperchromatic nuclei within a single cell. The cell may be so closely packed with nuclei that relatively little cytoplasm may remain visible (*Figs.* 2.56–58). This tight packing and the hyperchromatic nature of the nuclei help to differentiate such cells from osteoclasts (*Fig.* 2.57). Bizarre mitoses can be found in many of these giant polyploid cells (*Figs.* 2.56, 2.57 and 2.59). Enzyme

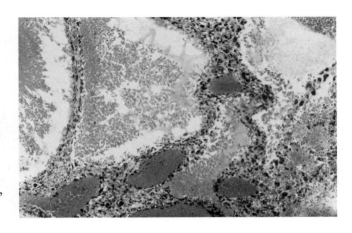

Fig. 2.49. **Telangiectatic osteosarcoma.** Low-power histological view of tumour, showing delicate septa of tumour transecting large aneurysmal vascular spaces. The general structure, but not the cellular composition, resembles aneurysmal bone cyst. (HE × 48.)

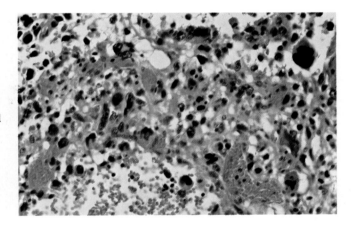

Fig. 2.50. **Telangiectatic osteosarcoma.** Histology: septum between aneurysmal spaces, showing pleomorphic anaplastic sarcoma, without any identifiable endothelial lining separating tumour from the aneurysmal blood spaces above and below. (HE × 192.)

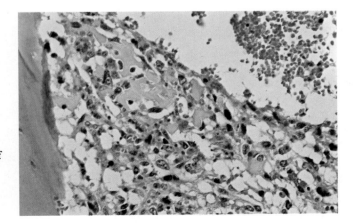

Fig. 2.51. **Telangiectatic osteosarcoma.** Histology of selected area showing production of tumour osteoid. Such areas may be few and far between. (HE × 192.)

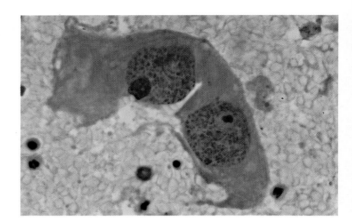

Fig. 2.52. **Telangiectatic osteosarcoma.** Smear showing bizarre tumour giant-cell with two huge nuclei with granular primitive chromatin structure. (HE × 480.)

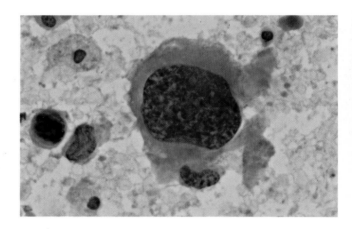

Fig. 2.53. **Telangiectatic osteosarcoma.** Smear showing bizarre giant cell with huge primitive nucleus. One of the smaller cells is in mitosis. (HE × 480.)

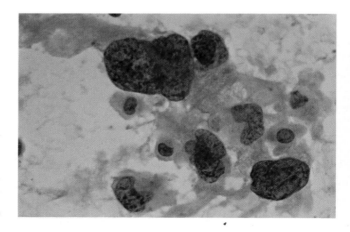

Fig. 2.54. **Telangiectatic osteosarcoma.** Smear showing pleomorphic tumour cells with giant nuclei. Several smaller tumour cells conform more closely in size to those found in less anaplastic osteosarcomas. (HE × 480.)

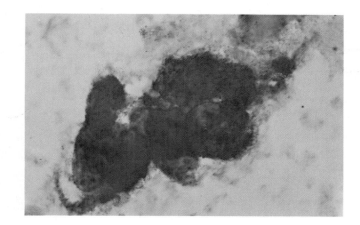

Fig. 2.55. **Telangiectatic osteosarcoma.** Smear: tumour giant-cells containing alkaline phosphatase in their cytoplasm. (Alkaline phosphatase preparation × 480.)

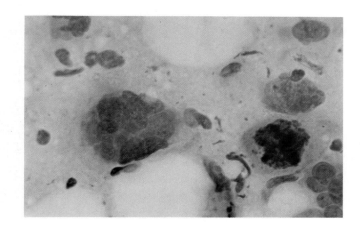

Fig. 2.56. **Anaplastic osteosarcoma.** Case 1. Smear showing tumour giant-cells with scanty cytoplasm and closely packed masses of nuclei. One of the giant tumour cells is in mitosis. (HE × 480.)

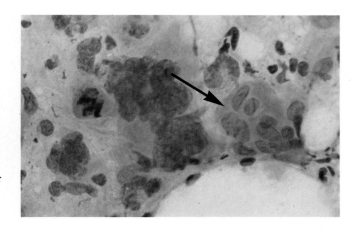

Fig. 2.57. **Anaplastic osteosarcoma.** Case 1. Smear: tumour giant-cells with closely packed masses of nuclei. Compare with osteoclast included in smear (arrowed). A cell in abnormal mitosis is also present. (HE × 480.)

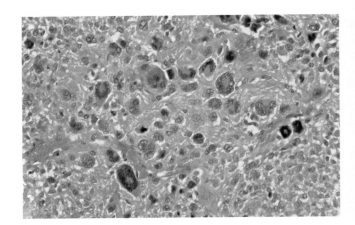

Fig. 2.58. **Anaplastic osteosarcoma.** Case 2. Histology: a pleomorphic sarcoma with abundant tumour giant-cells. (HE × 192.)

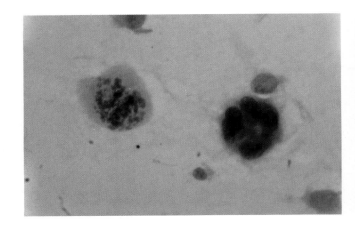

Fig. 2.59. **Anaplastic osteosarcoma.** Case 2. Smear showing two giant tumour cells, one with closely packed nuclei, the other in mitosis. (HE × 480.)

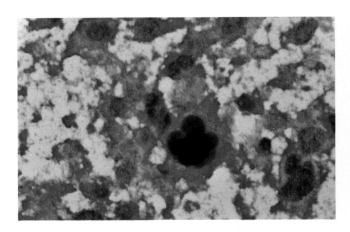

Fig. 2.60. **Anaplastic osteosarcoma.** Case 2. Smear: tumour cells rich in alkaline phosphatase, including several 'berry-like' multinucleate giant cells. (Alkaline phosphatase preparation × 480.)

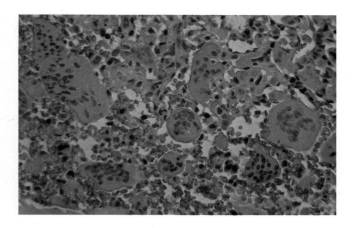

Fig. 2.61. **Anaplastic osteosarcoma.** Case 3. Histology of tumour at biopsy, showing over-abundance of osteoclasts, with individual osteosarcoma cells interspersed among them as 'stromal' cells. This was initially regarded as a malignant giant-cell tumour (malignant osteoclastoma) by the pathologists. The tumour was in the femoral diaphysis. (HE × 480.)

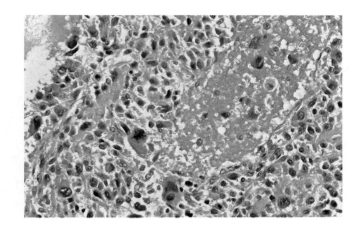

Fig. 2.62. **Anaplastic osteosarcoma.** Case 3. Histology of tumour at amputation, from telangiectatic part of the lesion. (HE × 192.)

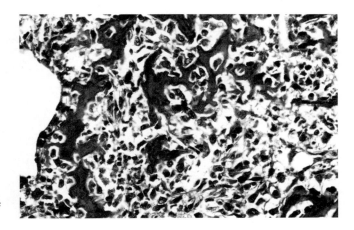

Fig. 2.63. **Anaplastic osteosarcoma.** Case 3. Histology at amputation, from osteoblastic part of the tumour. (HE × 192.)

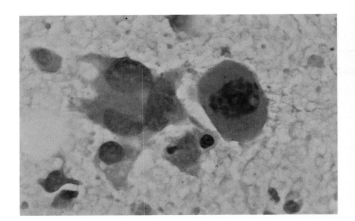

Fig. 2.64. **Anaplastic osteosarcoma.** Case 3. Representative field from cytological smear, showing two giant tumour cells, one in mitosis. (HE × 480.)

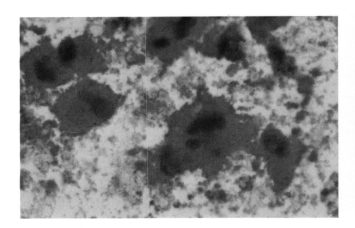

Fig. 2.65. **Anaplastic osteosarcoma.** Case 3. Smear: tumour cells rich in alkaline phosphatase. (Alkaline phosphatase preparation × 480.)

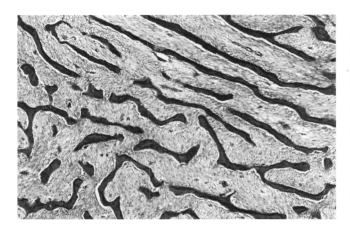

Fig. 2.66. **Parosteal osteosarcoma.** Typical histology showing fairly mature bone trabeculae formed in a low-grade fibro-cellular proliferate. The histological pattern was identical in the juxtacortical tumour and in its intra-osseous extension. (HE × 48.)

studies clarify the difference between the tumour giant cells and osteoclasts even more positively, since the former are alkaline phosphatase positive (*Fig.* 2.60), in sharp contrast with the osteoclastic giant cells which are acid phosphatase positive and alkaline phosphatase negative.

2. *Osteosarcoma in which there is an over-abundance of osteoclasts*

In rare instances of osteosarcoma, the tumour may be closely packed with osteoclasts so that the sarcoma cells appear almost as an incidental scattering among the osteoclasts. An example of this was seen in a 9-year-old child, and will illustrate the histological and cytological features of this variety, pinpointing the diagnostic difficulties that may arise from such a tumour. The patient presented with a tumour of the femur, which was biopsied at another hospital where the histological sections (*Fig.* 2.61) were interpreted as showing a malignant giant-cell tumour, i.e. a malignant osteoclastoma. The case was referred to this Registry and the pathologists on its panel also regarded it as a malignant giant-cell tumour, being guided in their diagnosis by the abundant osteoclasts, the plump malignant 'stromal' cells and the absence of tumour osteoid in the sampled material. The radiologists were adamantly against this diagnosis, insisting instead that the tumour was an osteosarcoma. Unfortunately, cytological smears were not available from the original biopsy. At subsequent amputation, the cytological (*Figs.* 2.64 and 2.65) and the histological (*Figs.* 2.62 and 2.63) findings were typical of osteosarcoma, parts showing a telangiectatic pattern (*Fig.* 2.62) and parts being osteoblastic (*Fig.* 2.63).

Parosteal osteosarcoma

Parosteal or juxtacortical osteosarcoma (*Fig.* 2.66) is characterized by its superficial origin on the outer surface of the cortex, its far better prognosis, and its characteristic histology showing relatively mature bone trabeculae embedded in a cellular fibrous or fibroblastic neoplastic proliferate. The example illustrated here showed infiltration of the underlying bone, but this is known to happen in about 10 % of juxtacortical osteosarcomas (van der Heul and von Ronnen, 1967) without adversely affecting its ultimate prognosis. Material excised from parosteal osteosarcoma is densely osteosclerotic and hence not particularly amenable to smearing, and we have no smears with which to demonstrate its cytological features. Like the more conventional osteosarcomas, the tumour cells—in this case fibroblast-like cells—are alkaline phosphatase positive, as demonstrable in cryostat sections.

References

Byers P.D. (1968) Solitary benign osteoblastic lesions of bone; osteoid osteoma and benign osteoblastoma. *Cancer 22*, 43.

Dahlin D.C. and Johnson E.W. jun. (1954) Giant osteoid osteoma. *J. Bone Joint Surg. 36-A*, 559.

Jaffe H.L. (1958) *Tumors and Tumorous Conditions of the Bones and Joints*. Philadelphia, Lea & Febiger, pp. 102, 526.

Lichtenstein L. (1956) Benign osteoblastoma. A category of osteoid- and bone-forming tumors other than classical osteoid osteoma which may be mistaken for giant-cell tumor or osteogenic sarcoma. *Cancer 9*, 1044.

Lichtenstein L. (1972) *Bone Tumors*, 4th ed. St Louis, Mosby, pp. 97–99, 112–115.

Mayer L. (1967) Malignant degeneration of so-called benign osteoblastoma. *Bull. Hosp. Joint Dis. 28*, 4.

Pochaczevsky R., Yen Y.M. and Sherman R.S. (1960) The roentgen appearance of benign osteoblastoma. *Radiology 75*, 429.

Schajowicz F. and Lemos C. (1970) Osteoid osteoma and osteoblastoma. Closely related entities of osteoblastic derivation. *Acta Orthop. Scand. 41*, 272.

Schajowicz F. and Lemos C. (1976) Malignant osteoblastoma. *J. Bone Joint Surg.* **58-B**, 202.

Spjut H.J., Dorfman H.D., Fechner R.E. and Ackerman L.V. (1971) *Tumors of Bone and Cartilage.* Washington D.C., Armed Forces Institute of Pathology, p. 120.

van der Heul R.O. and von Ronnen J.R. (1967) Juxtacortical osteosarcoma (diagnosis, differential diagnosis, treatment, and an analysis of 80 cases). *J. Bone Joint Surg.* **49-A**, 415.

Chapter 3

Cartilage Tumours and Chordoma

In this chapter chordoma will be considered in addition to the cartilage-forming tumours because it may occasionally have a chondroid matrix and may even be mistaken for chondrosarcoma. Chondromyxoid fibroma is also considered in this chapter because it is not infrequently confused with chondrosarcoma; furthermore, it is probably more related to chondroid tumours than to fibromas. Chondroblastoma will be dealt with in Chapter 5, with giant-cell-containing lesions, because it is often rich in osteoclasts and requires differentiation from giant-cell tumour of bone.

Normal cartilage and benign cartilage tumours with well-formed mature cartilaginous matrix are difficult to smear because their constituent cells are imprisoned in a firmly set gel and cannot be easily dislodged. When mature cartilaginous tissue is firmly crushed between the forceps during the smearing process, only a small number of dislodged free cells will be deposited on the slide and most of the smeared material will consist of shredded cartilage matrix with the chondrocytes still trapped therein. This difficulty in smearing is, in itself, a useful indication of the benignity of such lesions. In chondrosarcomas, the matrix tends to be less mature and more myxoid and such tumours usually yield perfectly adequate smears with abundant tumour cells.

Mucoid material is spread onto the slide in the preparation of smears from chondroid tumours, so that the background stains metachromatically with Taylor's blue (*Figs*. 3.17, 3.31 and 3.35). This background metachromasia is helpful in distinguishing chondroid tumours from certain non-chondroid tumours with which they may be confused, for instance some cases of chondroblastoma from giant-cell tumour of bone. Glycogen is usually present in normal chondrocytes and the more differentiated chondroid tumour cells (*Fig*. 3.3). Alkaline phosphatase is present in the chondrocytes at the zone of ossification of the epiphysial plate (Gomori, 1939), and evolutionary endochondral ossification may be found to some degree in many cartilaginous tumours, both benign and malignant. For this reason, it would be surprising if some alkaline phosphatase activity were not to be seen in cartilage tumours, despite the observation of Remagen et al. (1976) that cartilaginous tumours are poor in phosphatase activity. In our own experience a proportion of alkaline phosphatase positive cartilage cells can be seen in smears of enchondromas and chondrosarcomas (*Fig*. 3.16). We have already referred to this phenomenon in Chapter 2 (p. 19); nevertheless, in such cases the cytomorphology is sufficiently explicit for chondrosarcoma not to be confused with chondroblastic osteosarcoma.

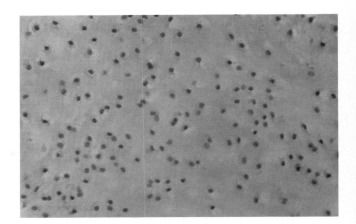

Fig. 3.1. **Enchondroma.**
Histology: fully mature
tumour with uniformly
small chondrocytes having
small dark condensed
nuclei. (HE × 192.)

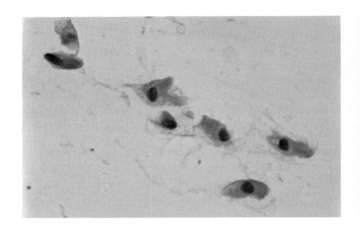

Fig. 3.2. **Enchondroma.**
Same case as in *Fig.* 3.1.
Smear showing
chondrocytes with small
mature condensed nuclei.
(HE × 480.)

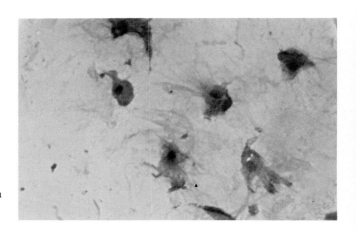

Fig. 3.3. **Enchondroma.**
Glycogen is demonstrable in
the chondrocytes.
(PAS × 480.)

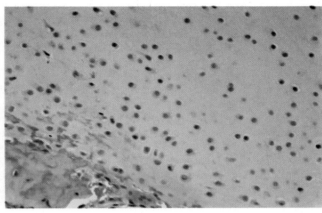

Fig. 3.4. **Enchondroma.**
Another case. Histology is
essentially similar to that
seen in *Fig*. 3.1, but
numbers of chondrocytes
show less condensed nuclei.
There was no evidence of
cortical or intertrabecular
infiltration in any part of the
tumour. (HE × 192.)

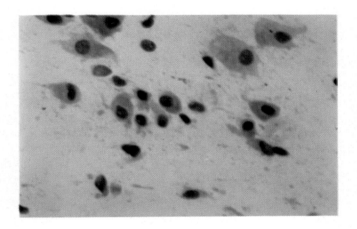

Fig. 3.5. **Enchondroma.**
Same case as in *Fig*. 3.4.
Smear showing some
variation in nuclear size.
Some nuclei are small and
fully condensed, others are
larger and show only partial
condensation of chromatin.
Binucleate cells were very
rare. (HE × 480.)

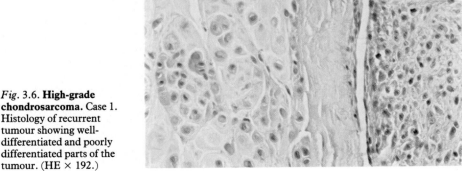

Fig. 3.6. **High-grade
chondrosarcoma.** Case 1.
Histology of recurrent
tumour showing well-
differentiated and poorly
differentiated parts of the
tumour. (HE × 192.)

CHONDROMA

The cytological characteristics of benign cartilaginous proliferations are similar whether one examines an enchondroma, ecchondroma, soft-tissue chondroma or the cartilage cap of an osteochondroma. We will therefore confine our illustrations to material from enchondromas.

Histologically, enchondroma presents fairly uniform small cartilage cells with small round dark condensed nuclei (*Figs.* 3.1 and 3.4). Binucleate cells are scanty or absent and their nuclei, like those of the mononucleate cells, are small and dark. Enchondroma grows slowly and expansively on a broad front. The osseous tissue it approaches is not infiltrated but is gradually removed by osteoclastic activity, and a new cortical shell is eventually formed beyond the ultimate limits of the tumour. Calcification and evolutionary ossification may occur in the substance of the tumour. In some cases, trabeculae of the original host bone may be found apparently embedded in cartilage, because of cartilage rests which have developed *pari passu* with the bone itself. Such trabeculae are intact, not disrupted or partly destroyed, and are separated from the cartilage by its perichondrium. When trabeculae of host bone become sequestrated in invading chondrosarcoma, the tumour cartilage abuts directly on the bone trabeculae and the latter show evidence of irregular resorption and destruction. The matrix of a benign cartilage tumour is normally mature and well-formed, for which reason it is difficult to make smears from it. Some chondromas have a less rigid and more mucoid matrix and these provide better smears (illustrations below are from such cases).

Smears from benign cartilage tumours show small cells (*Figs.* 3.2 and 3.5) with glycogen in their cytoplasm (*Fig.* 3.3) and have small round or ovoid mature condensed dark nuclei. In actively growing enchondromas (*Figs.* 3.4, 3.5) a number of chondrocytes may have nuclei larger than is usual with indolent mature chondromas. Binucleate cells are rare; multinucleate cells are absent. Like all chondroid tumours, the background of their smears stains metachromatically with Taylor's blue. Small numbers of cells may be alkaline phosphatase positive.

CHONDROSARCOMA

The diagnosis of chondrosarcoma may present formidable, and at times seemingly insurmountable, difficulties (Dahlin, 1967). Perhaps more than any other bone tumour, its diagnosis requires careful assessment of all clinical, radiological, histological and, not least, cytological information.

The importance of paying attention to cytological detail, particularly of the cell nuclei, in examining histological sections of cartilage tumours has been stressed by most authors. Lichtenstein and Jaffe (1943) consider that a cartilage tumour should not be regarded as benign if, when viable non-calcifying areas are examined, it shows, even in scattered fields, (1) many cells with plump nuclei, (2) more than an occasional cell with two such nuclei, and especially (3) giant cartilage cells with large single or multiple nuclei or with clumps of chromatin.

It is our view and experience that the cytological detail of such tumours can be optimally studied in smears and we are convinced that these provide collateral information of significant diagnostic importance in their assessment. Salzer-Kuntschik (1976) has come to a similar conclusion, that 'the histologically recognizable degree of malignancy of chondrosarcoma can be evaluated better with the cytologic than with the histologic technic'.

In the literature most histological accounts of chondrosarcoma give pride of place to a description of the cytological abnormalities and largely ignore consideration of histological evidence of invasiveness in relation to the host bone. In examining histological sections we specifically look for such evidence and we must stress its reliability and importance. A chondrosarcoma, however well-differentiated it may be, will infiltrate between the trabeculae of host bone, intimately abut on them without the intervention of any fibrous perichondrium, disrupt and eventually encase their remnants. This disruption of the bone trabeculae is indirect, through osteoclastic activity in the host tissue. Nevertheless, where tumour abuts directly on eroded trabecular bone, usually no osteoclasts are identifiable along the line of contact. The inference is that the osteoclasts have been destroyed by the invading tumour and osteoclasis thereby terminated, so that the disrupted trabeculae undergo no further resorption but remain embedded within the tumour (*Figs.* 3.13, 3.20 and 3.24). With benign cartilage tumours bone is similarly eaten away by osteoclasts, but the latter are not prematurely overtaken by the tumour and have sufficient time to complete their task; the bone disappears beyond the advancing edge of the tumour and does not remain to be sequestrated within the tumour. Chondrosarcoma will infiltrate the normal corticalis (*Fig.* 3.19) and gain access to the extra-cortical tissues. When a hitherto benign cartilage tumour undergoes malignant change, the evolutionary bone previously formed through endochondral ossification of its matrix may similarly become invaded, disrupted and engulfed (*Fig.* 3.13). The adventitious shell of bone formed around an old enchondroma will become eroded and perforated by chondrosarcoma (*Fig.* 3.11) when the latter supervenes, as it may, many decades later.

Four cases of conventional chondrosarcoma will be described to illustrate the broad range of its histology and cytology.

Case 1. High-grade chondrosarcoma.
The patient was first seen in 1965, at the age of 51, with pain and limitation of movement of the right shoulder and was then thought to have supraspinatus tendinitis. No radiological changes were then present. The symptoms persisted and in 1967 X-rays showed a destructive lesion of the head of the humerus with cortical perforation. Biopsy and subsequent resection of the upper end of the humerus showed a well-differentiated chondrosarcoma occupying the medullary cavity and breaking out through the corticalis to produce a cuff of tumour around the anatomical neck of the humerus. Five years later, in 1972, a large local recurrence was removed and showed (*Figs.* 3.6 and 3.7), in addition to some residual well-differentiated chondrosarcoma, a poorly differentiated tumour with abundant mitoses. Further local recurrences developed and the patient died in 1973, without demonstrable pulmonary metastases. Palliative radiotherapy was given only after the 1972 recurrence, so that the progression to anaplasia cannot be attributed to irradiation.

Cytological preparations from the 1972 recurrence show cells derived from the different areas of the tumour. 'Ring chondroblasts' (*Fig.* 3.8), derived from the well-differentiated part of the tumour, are seen as individual cells or small groups of cells within their own individual matrix. This is in contrast with benign chondromas in which the chondrocytes, when not dislodged from the cartilaginous matrix, are seen encased in a communal matrix. The nuclei are small, perhaps no larger than those of a chondroma, but unlike the latter still show relatively uncondensed nuclear chromatin. Cells derived from the anaplastic part of the chondrosarcoma (*Figs.* 3.9 and 3.10) have open primitive nuclei many times larger than those of a chondroma, indeed larger than those of low-grade chondrosarcomas, and mitoses can be found with relative ease, unlike medium-grade or low-grade chondrosarcomas in which mitoses are rare or absent. In this case, alkaline phosphatase was absent in all the tumour cells, whether well-differentiated or anaplastic.

Case 2. Medium-grade chondrosarcoma.
The patient, aged 74, had had a swelling over the dorso-medial surface of the proximal phalanx of the left great toe for 50 years. During recent years it had doubled in size and had been giving discomfort from a corn overlying it. It was clinically thought to be an osteochondroma and was locally excised in 1976.

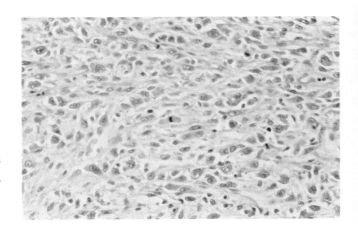

Fig. 3.7. **High-grade
chondrosarcoma.** Case 1.
Histology: undifferentiated
sarcoma with abundant
mitoses. Mitoses are rare or
absent in medium or low-
grade chondrosarcomas.
(HE × 192.)

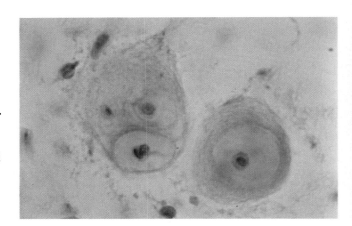

Fig. 3.8. **Chondrosarcoma.**
Case 1. Smear showing well
differentiated tumour cells
derived from the low-grade
part of the tumour. One cell
is surrounded by its own
individual matrix. The
nuclei are small but only
partly condensed.
(HE × 480.)

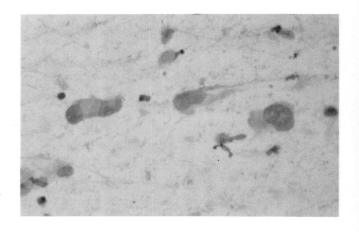

Fig. 3.9. **High-grade
chondrosarcoma.** Case 1.
Smear showing
undifferentiated tumour
cells with large open nuclei;
one of them is binucleate.
(HE × 480.)

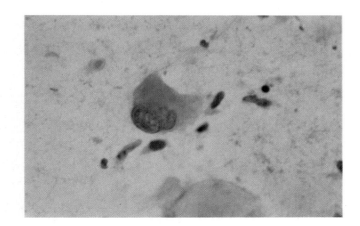

Fig. 3.10. **High-grade chondrosarcoma.** Case 1. Smear from poorly differentiated part of tumour, showing a large binucleate tumour cell. (HE × 480.)

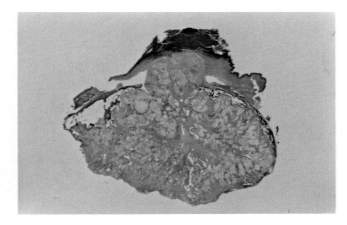

Fig. 3.11. **Medium-grade chondrosarcoma.** Case 2. Mounted section showing extension of tumour beyond cortical shell of old chondroma. (Masson's trichrome × 2·4.)

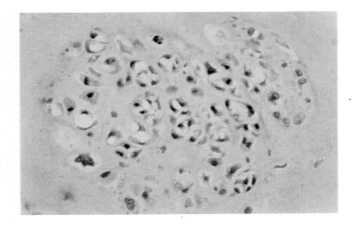

Fig. 3.12. **Medium-grade chondrosarcoma.** Case 2. Histology of tumour. Numbers of tumour cells have open nucleolated nuclei. A multinucleate tumour cell is seen (below left). A field such as this could be dismissed as showing an ordinary chondroma on superficial examination. Indeed, on histological criteria this was diagnosed as a low-grade, not a medium-grade, chondrosarcoma. (HE × 192.)

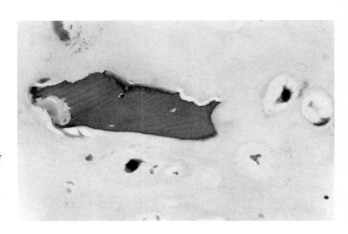

Fig. 3.13. **Medium-grade chondrosarcoma.** Case 2. Histology showing a disrupted remnant of trabecular bone embedded in tumour cartilage. Although the cartilage here is relatively acellular, the field is quite characteristic of an invasive cartilage tumour and provides histological evidence of chondrosarcoma. (HE × 192.)

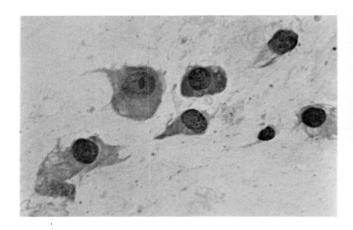

Fig. 3.14. **Medium-grade chondrosarcoma.** Case 2. Smear: group of tumour cells showing appreciable nuclear pleomorphism. Nuclei primitive and stippled; obvious nucleolus is present in largest nucleus. (HE × 480.)

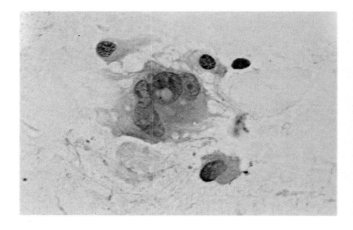

Fig. 3.15. **Medium-grade chondrosarcoma.** Case 2. Smear showing multinucleate tumour cell with large primitive nucleolated nuclei. Several small tumour cells show only partial nuclear condensation and some variation in nuclear size. (HE × 480.)

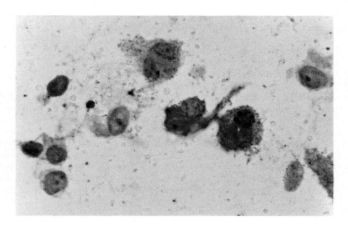

Fig. 3.16. **Medium-grade chondrosarcoma.** Case 2. Smear: a small proportion of the tumour cells contain alkaline phosphatase; these are relatively more mature than the enzyme-negative cells. It is believed that this enzyme activity is analogous to that seen in maturing cells of the normal epiphysial plate. (Alkaline phosphatase preparation × 480.)

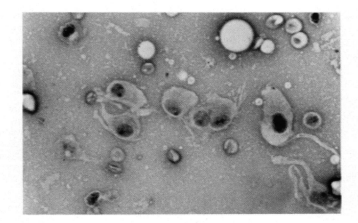

Fig. 3.17. **Medium-grade chondrosarcoma.** Case 2. Metachromasia of the background. This is a feature of all chondroid tumours. (Taylor's blue × 480.)

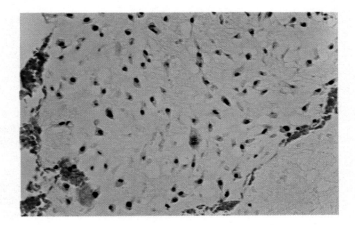

Fig. 3.18. **Medium-grade chondrosarcoma.** Case 3. Histology of biopsy material, showing chondromyxoid tumour, sometimes confused with chondromyxoid fibroma. (HE × 192.)

The specimen showed a partly ossified cartilage tumour with a thin shell of mature bone surrounding its outer aspect. Tumour had broken out through the dome of this shell (*Fig.* 3.11), causing ulceration and scabbing of the overlying skin. Part of the tumour cartilage was firm and well-formed, parts were quite soft, gelatinous and pinkish in colour.

Histology showed the features expected from a chondrosarcoma, with obvious cellular and nuclear pleomorphism (*Fig.* 3.12) and there was evidence of invasive behaviour: (1) infiltration, disruption and sequestration of trabecular bone (*Fig.* 3.13) which, in this case, is clearly bone which had formed through past ossification of the matrix of a pre-existing chondroma, and (2) penetration of the cortical shell, with extension into the adjoining soft tissues (*Fig.* 3.11). On histological examination, this was reported as a low-grade chondrosarcoma, because the precise cytological detail was not fully recognized from the sections.

Smears (*Figs.* 3.14 and 3.15), prepared with great ease, show cells with large primitive nuclei, having open finely stippled chromatin and prominent nucleoli. Binucleate and multinucleate cells (*Fig.* 3.15) can be found. No mitoses were seen; their absence or scarcity is a feature of all but undifferentiated chondrosarcomas. Alkaline phosphatase is present in about 20 % of the tumour cells (*Fig.* 3.16), not all to a marked degree, and the background is metachromatic with Taylor's blue (*Fig.* 3.17).

Case 3. Medium-grade chondrosarcoma.
A 49-year-old man presented with pain in the left shoulder and X-rays showed altered architecture in the humeral cortex, with periosteal reaction and some trabeculation. Biopsy in 1976, at another hospital, was reported as containing myxomatous areas with stellate and fusiform cells, and chondromyxoid fibroma was suggested as a definite possibility. Pathologists at another hospital thought that it was either a chondroma or a chondromyxoid fibroma. A repeat biopsy was performed and examined at this Laboratory, where it was diagnosed as a chondrosarcoma of medium grade, in parts producing chondroid, in others a loose myxoid matrix (*Fig.* 3.18). There was obvious infiltration of the Haversian canals in the corticalis (*Fig.* 3.19), another clear evidence of malignancy. A forequarter amputation was performed and showed an extensive chondrosarcoma occupying much of the humeral cavity and intimately infiltrating the corticalis to produce numerous subperiosteal nodules of tumour. The manner in which a chondrosarcoma infiltrates, disrupts and sequestrates the trabeculae of host bone is clearly shown in *Fig.* 3.20.

Smears, prepared with great ease, show cells several times larger than the chondrocytes of an indolent chondroma, with correspondingly larger nuclei and a relative abundance of binucleate cells (*Figs.* 3.21 and 3.22); an occasional giant cell with large nucleolated nucleus can also be seen. The background of the smear is richly metachromatic with Taylor's blue. Alkaline phosphatase can be demonstrated in about 40 % of the tumour cells, fairly richly in perhaps half of them. Despite the presence of alkaline phosphatase in so many cells, the cytomorphology of this chondrosarcoma is manifestly different from that of chondroblastic osteosarcoma, so that no diagnostic confusion can possibly arise.

Case 4. Low-grade chondrosarcoma.
A 47-year-old woman had had pain in the left wrist since 1967. In 1969 X-rays showed widening and 'cystic' change in the left trapezium and this was curetted out in another country, with the incorrect—presumably non-histological—diagnosis of aneurysmal bone cyst. Recurrence in 1973 was again curetted out, this time with a diagnosis of osteochondroma. Pain and swelling persisted and she sought surgical treatment in this country. Biopsy and radical surgery showed a cellular low-grade chondrosarcoma (*Figs.* 3.23 and 3.24). Tumour from the trapezium had invaded and infiltrated the adjoining trapezoid and the base of the second metacarpal. There was evidence of invasion, tumour disrupting and encasing bone trabeculae (*Fig.* 3.24) and penetrating the cortical shell.

Cytological smears (*Figs.* 3.25 and 3.26) show large open nuclei, some with nucleoli, and fair numbers of binucleate cells. A comparison with the cytomorphology of Case 3 shows substantial similarities between these two cases. In this case, no alkaline phosphatase was demonstrable in any of the tumour cells.

A comparison of the nuclear size in various benign and malignant cartilaginous tumours is given in black-and-white outlines, drawn at the same magnification.

The difficulties in the diagnosis of chondrosarcoma fall broadly into three groups.

1. *Chondroblastic osteosarcoma.* In the past, before the true nature of chondroblastic osteosarcoma was fully recognized, this variety of osteosarcoma was often misdiagnosed as chondrosarcoma. Among the chondrosarcomas classified in the

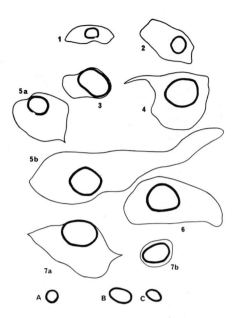

Line drawings of representative cells from cartilage tumours. Osteoclast and small lymphocyte nuclei are also given for comparison.

These and all other line drawings in this volume have been drawn at the same magnification.

1. Enchondroma, quiescent (cell from *Fig.* 3.2).
2. Enchondroma, active and cellular, from Ollier's disease in an adolescent patient (one of the larger cells from *Fig.* 3.5).
3. High-grade chondrosarcoma (cell from *Fig.* 3.9).
4. Medium-grade chondrosarcoma (cell from *Fig.* 3.14).
5. Medium-grade chondrosarcoma, average and large cells from the same patient:
    5a: Average-sized nucleus (cell from *Fig.* 3.21).
    5b: Large nucleus (cell from *Fig.* 3.22).
6. Low-grade chondrosarcoma (cell from *Fig.* 3.25).
7. 'Chondroblastic sarcoma' (cells from *Fig.* 3.30):
    7a: Large nucleus.
    7b: Average-sized nucleus.
A. Nucleus of small lymphocyte.
B. Nucleus of juvenile osteoclast.
C. Nucleus of mature osteoclast.

Nuclei of chondrosarcomas of all grades are appreciably larger than those of enchondromas. The malignancy of a smear from a cartilage tumour, and its grade, is not assessed on nuclear size alone; other features, particularly chromatin structure and presence of multinucleate cells, must be taken into account.

earlier years of this Registry were half a dozen or so chondroblastic osteosarcomas, which have since been re-classified. Even today, the danger of misdiagnosing chondroblastic osteosarcoma as chondrosarcoma remains, particularly with histological examination of limited biopsy material and disregard of clinical and radiological data.

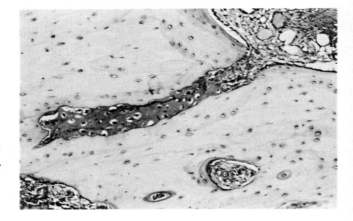

Fig. 3.19. **Medium-grade chondrosarcoma.** Case 3. Histology of biopsy material, showing extension of cartilage tumour into the corticalis—clear evidence of invasiveness, hence of chondrosarcoma. (Taylor's blue × 77.)

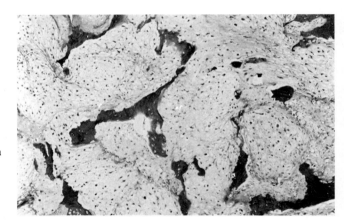

Fig. 3.20. **Medium-grade chondrosarcoma.** Case 3. Histology of intramedullary chondrosarcoma showing disruption and sequestration of bone trabeculae within the cartilage tumour— another typical evidence of chondrosarcoma. (HE × 48.)

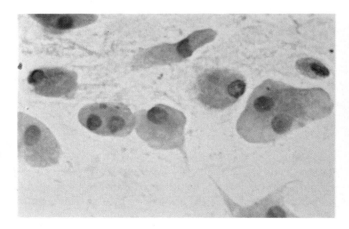

Fig. 3.21. **Medium-grade chondrosarcoma.** Case 3. Smear showing tumour cells with only partially condensed nuclear chromatin; fairly frequent binucleate cells. (HE × 480.)

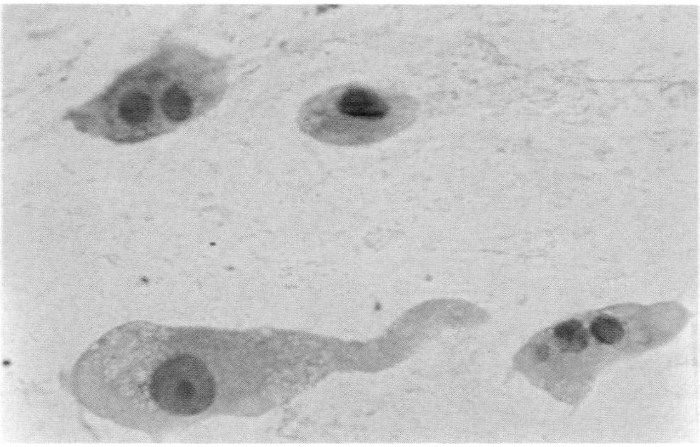

Fig. 3.22. **Medium-grade chondrosarcoma.** Case 3. Smear showing four tumour cells, including two binucleate cells and a large tadpole-shaped cell with large nucleolated nucleus. Such large cells were relatively rare in the smears from this case. (HE × 480.)

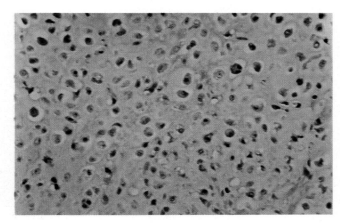

Fig. 3.23. **Low-grade chondrosarcoma.** Case 4. Histology: cartilage tumour with relatively uncondensed nuclei and occasional binucleate cells. This type of tumour could be dismissed as a 'cellular chondroma'. (HE × 192.)

Fig. 3.24. **Low-grade chondrosarcoma.** Case 4. Histology: bone trabeculae irregularly eroded, disrupted and sequestrated in tumour cartilage, providing evidence of the invasive nature of the tumour. The invasiveness was also evinced macroscopically by the fact that tumour had extended into two other adjoining bones. (HE × 48.)

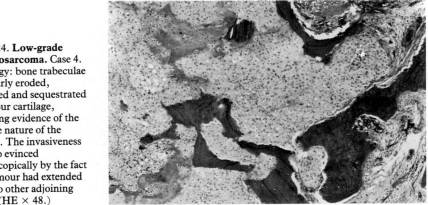

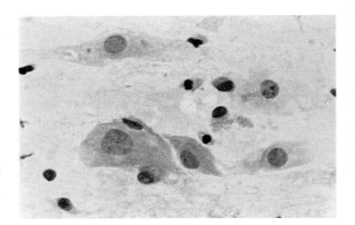

Fig. 3.25. **Low-grade chondrosarcoma.** Case 4. Smear showing variations in cell and nuclear size; some are condensed and small, others are large and uncondensed. (HE × 480.)

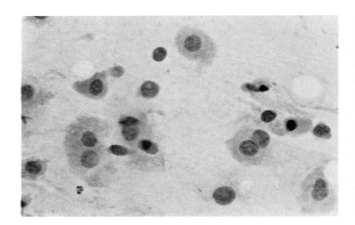

Fig. 3.26. **Low-grade chondrosarcoma.** Case 4. Smear showing two binucleate cells, similar to those present in *Case 3* (*Figs.* 3.21 and 3.22). (HE × 480.)

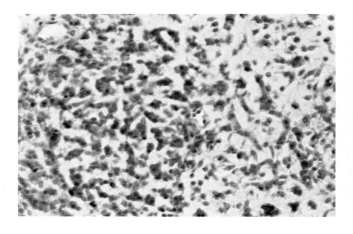

Fig. 3.27. **'Chondroblastic sarcoma'.** Histology of tumour: strands of ovoid cells in a myxoid stroma. Osteoclast-type giant cells were absent in all fields; osteoclasts would be expected in benign chondroblastoma. (HE × 192.)

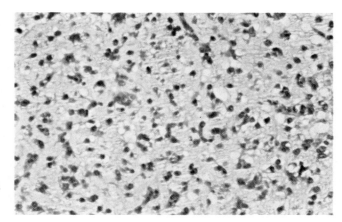

Fig. 3.28. **'Chondroblastic sarcoma'.** Histology of tumour from less cellular areas: abundant myxoid stroma with occasional cords and nests of tumour cells. (HE × 192.)

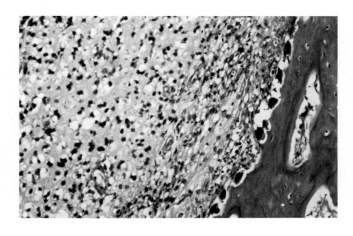

Fig. 3.29. **'Chondroblastic sarcoma'.** Histology: behaviour of tumour in relation to corticalis is *not* infiltrative. The cortex is being eroded on a wide front, and the osteoclasts have not been 'overtaken' and destroyed by the tumour. This feature indicates that this is not an invasive tumour. (HE × 120.)

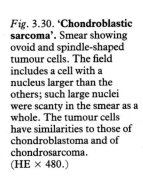

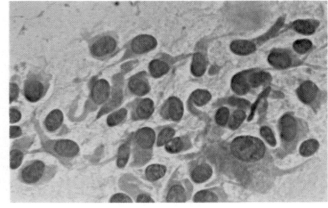

Fig. 3.30. **'Chondroblastic sarcoma'.** Smear showing ovoid and spindle-shaped tumour cells. The field includes a cell with a nucleus larger than the others; such large nuclei were scanty in the smear as a whole. The tumour cells have similarities to those of chondroblastoma and of chondrosarcoma. (HE × 480.)

The great majority of chondrosarcomas are well or moderately differentiated tumours, of low or medium-grade malignancy, and their cytomorphology is quite different from that of chondroblastic osteosarcoma. Their smears show smaller and less primitive nuclei than does chondroblastic osteosarcoma, and mitoses are absent or scarce. The fact that some such chondrosarcomas may contain alkaline phosphatase in a variable proportion of the tumour cells will not, therefore, create any problems in cytodiagnosis. Poorly differentiated chondrosarcomas are relatively rare. During the period of 8 years in which we have used cytological smears, only one such tumour has been recorded in this Registry and this proved singularly devoid of alkaline phosphatase.

2. *Chondromyxoid fibroma.* Chondromyxoid fibroma may be misdiagnosed as chondrosarcoma, and we still come across such instances. It is even more likely these days that chondrosarcoma may be mistakenly diagnosed as chondromyxoid fibroma. Smears of chondromyxoid fibroma contain scattered osteoclasts, which is not a feature of chondrosarcomas, as well as myxoid, fibrocytoid and chondroid cells. Some of the latter may be binucleate or multinucleate but their nuclei are usually condensed or 'smudgy' and smaller than those of chondrosarcoma.

3. *Chondroma.* The greatest difficulty arises in the differentiation of low-grade chondrosarcoma, even of medium-grade chondrosarcoma, from chondroma. Our understanding of low-grade chondrosarcoma has been decidedly inadequate, and much mythology and dogmatism still persist in confusing the issue. For instance, there is the belief that a cartilage tumour in the hands and feet must be benign and that cartilage tumours of the shoulder and pelvic girdles must be considered malignant, irrespective of the histology. In this Registry the diagnosis of malignancy in the past was often based not on the histology but on clinical criteria—a cartilage tumour which showed growth activity in later life and caused pain was considered probably malignant. This clinical judgement is usually sound and relevant; nevertheless, confirmatory histological and cytological evidence should be, and we now believe *is*, equally reliable. Otherwise, we will still continue to talk about 'histologically benign' but 'clinically malignant' cartilage tumours. The histological and cytological differences between chondrosarcoma and chondroma has, we hope, been convincingly demonstrated in the cases illustrated above. Tumours with borderline cytological characteristics and without histological evidence of invasiveness are, however, bound to arise and are best regarded as 'borderline cartilage tumours'.

It is important to explain our concept of malignancy in relation to low-grade chondrosarcoma, in that this is essentially limited to local invasiveness, with negligible metastatic risk. By and large, low-grade chondrosarcomas behave as locally invasive tumours which, when inadequately removed, will continue to grow and will eventually 'recur'. Inadequacy of removal, recurrence and death from local invasion is particularly experienced in such inaccessible sites as the pelvis. The emphasis on the alleged benignity of peripheral cartilage tumours may, in part, be a reflection of their accessibility and curability by local amputation. We fully concur with Gottschalk and Smith (1963) that too great a reliance must not be placed on the location of a cartilage tumour and we agree with Lichtenstein (1972) that digital chondrosarcomas may have been underdiagnosed in the past. During the past 8 years, using our cytological and histological criteria, 8 of our chondrosarcomas were in the distal extremities beyond the wrist and ankle joints.

MESENCHYMAL CHONDROSARCOMA AND CHONDROBLASTIC SARCOMA

Lichtenstein and Bernstein (1959) recorded examples of unusual cartilaginous tumours and a more recent account of these has been given by Lichtenstein (1972). Among these are two rather characteristic, but rare, tumours: mesenchymal chondrosarcoma and 'chondroblastic sarcoma'.

Mesenchymal chondrosarcoma is a highly cellular primitive-looking tumour with rounded or stubby spindle cells which would not be readily recognizable as of cartilaginous origin were it not for the fact that foci of differentiated cartilage can be found within the tumour. Sooner or later, the tumour involves many other bones, probably as a reflection of a multicentric origin rather than of metastasis. No example of this tumour has been recorded in this Registry and we cannot, therefore, illustrate its cytology.

'Chondroblastic sarcoma'. Lichtenstein (1972) regards this as a low-grade chondrosarcoma, different biologically and cytologically from conventional chondrosarcoma, showing a consistent tendency to insidious local extension, but with little or no disposition towards early metastasis.

We have recently seen a probable example of such a tumour. A 24-year-old woman presented with one year's history of pain in the shoulder, and X-rays showed an expansile lesion in the proximal humerus which was thought to be a giant-cell tumour. Biopsy and subsequent resection showed an unusual chondroblastic tumour (*Figs*. 3.27 and 3.28) composed of strands or cords of ovoid cells growing in a myxoid matrix. In parts the tumour cells lay singly or in small nests separated by abundant matrix; in others, they were more closely packed together and showed a tendency to be spindle-shaped, with fair numbers of mitoses. There was no infiltration of the intertrabecular spaces or the Haversian canals. The tumour had grown expansively (*Fig*. 3.29) eroding the cortex on a broad front, with formation of a secondary shell of bone beyond. In places, this shell was deficient and tumour had briefly extended into the soft tissues beyond.

Cytological smears (*Figs*. 3.30 and 3.31) show a richly metachromatic background with round, ovoid and fusiform cells which bear some resemblance both to chondrosarcoma cells and to the cells of chondroblastoma. No significant nuclear pleomorphism is present; the nuclei are of relatively similar size and only very occasional cells with larger nuclei can be found. Binucleate or multinucleate tumour cells are absent, as are osteoclasts. Alkaline phosphatase is not demonstrable in the tumour cells.

Giant-cell tumour, which had been suspected clinically, could be immediately ruled out by the cytology. Conventional chondrosarcoma was ruled out on both cytological and histological criteria: even low-grade chondrosarcomas show fairly abundant binucleate cells and present histological evidence of invasive activity. The tumour did not show the usual features expected in chondroblastoma and was lacking in osteoclasts. Two other possible diagnoses were proffered by other pathologists: chondroblastic osteosarcoma and mesenchymal chondrosarcoma. The tumour was devoid of alkaline phosphatase and showed none of the pleomorphic cytomorphology found in chondroblastic osteosarcoma, which was therefore ruled out. We do not consider that the histology of this tumour quite conforms to that of mesenchymal chondrosarcoma, as described and illustrated in the literature, although we cannot firmly rule out that diagnosis.

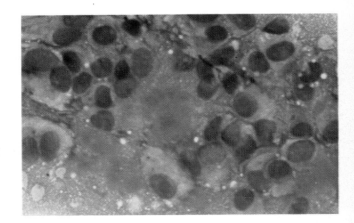

Fig. 3.31. **'Chondroblastic sarcoma'.** Smear showing metachromasia of the background. (Taylor's blue × 480.)

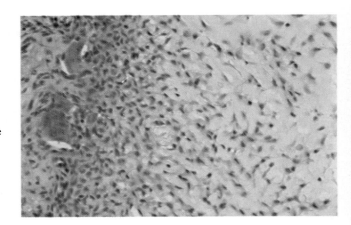

Fig. 3.32. **Chondromyxoid fibroma.** Typical histology: field showing part of a lobule with cellular periphery on the left. As the centre of the lobule is approached the amount of fibromyxoid matrix progressively increases. Osteoclasts are present along the periphery of the lobule. (HE × 192.)

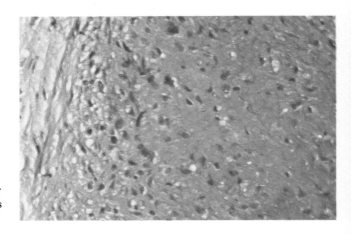

Fig. 3.33. **Chondromyxoid fibroma.** Histological section showing progressive increase in metachromatic matrix towards the centre of the tumour lobule. (Taylor's blue × 192.)

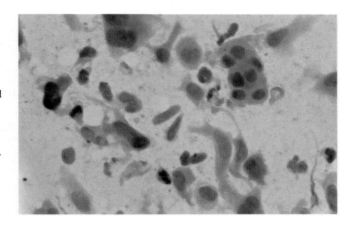

Fig. 3.34. **Chondromyxoid fibroma.** Typical smear showing an admixture of cell types, including an osteoclast, stellate myxoid cells, fusiform fibrocytoid cells and chondroid cells with eosinophilic cytoplasm. Some of the latter have double or lobulated nuclei; the latter are 'smudgy' or dark and condensed. (HE × 480.)

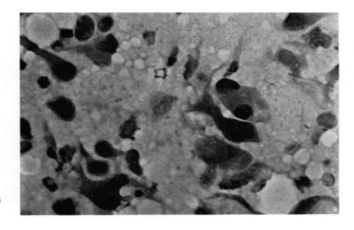

Fig. 3.35. **Chondromyxoid fibroma.** Smear showing metachromasia of the background. This is a feature of all chondroid tumours; it helps differentiate osteoclast-rich smears of chondromyxoid fibroma from giant-cell tumour and non-ossifying fibroma which may also be rich in osteoclasts. (Taylor's blue × 480.)

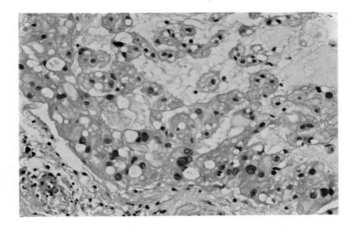

Fig. 3.36. **Chordoma.** Typical histological pattern. Large epithelioid cells, many with large vacuoles or blisters, tending to be arranged in cords in a mucinous stroma. Variable nuclear pleomorphism is usually present. (HE × 192.)

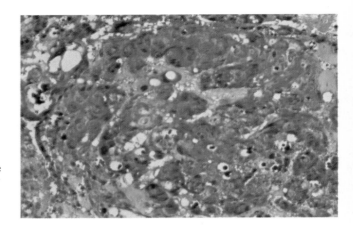

Fig. 3.37. **Chordoma.**
Histology: cytoplasm of the
tumour cells is rich in
glycogen. No glycogen is
present in the vacuoles.
(PAS × 192.)

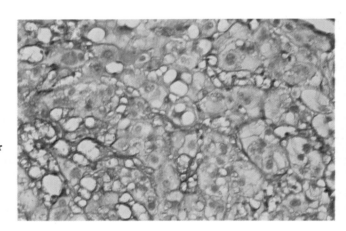

Fig. 3.38. **Chordoma.**
Histology: metachromatic
mucin is demonstrable
between the cords of tumour
cells. Mucin is also seen in
the cytoplasm of some cells.
Some of the vacuoles
apparently do not contain
mucin. (Taylor's
blue × 192.)

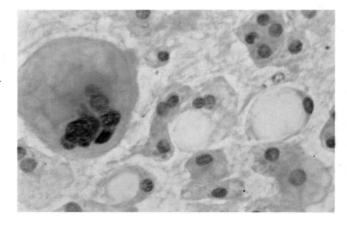

Fig. 3.39. **Chordoma.**
Typical smear from
chordoma, including a
multinucleate tumour giant-
cell. Three physaliphorous
cells with large single
vacuoles are present; these
may often be much larger
than shown here. Cells
without vacuoles appear
much smaller,
morphologically resembling
the cells of low-grade
chondrosarcoma.
(HE × 480.)

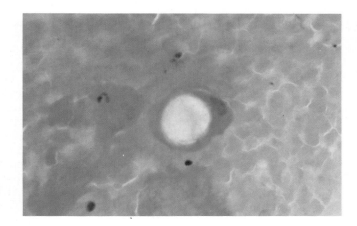

Fig. 3.40. Chordoma.
Smear: physaliphorous cell
with glycogen in its
cytoplasm. (PAS × 480.)

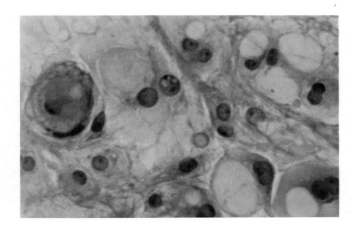

Fig. 3.41. Chordoma.
Smear: cluster of chordoma
cells, many with large
vacuoles. Some of these
vacuoles are moderately
metachromatic, others
faintly so. One large cell
contains clusters of small
vacuoles with
metachromatic mucin. A
few non-vacuolated cells
contain early demilunes of
mucin. (Taylor's
blue × 480.)

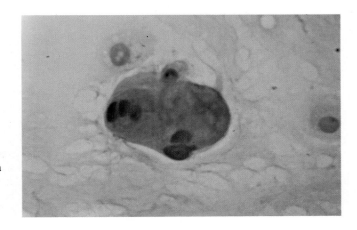

Fig. 3.42. Chordoma.
Smear showing a cluster of
chordoma cells, including a
binucleate cell with large
vacuole containing
metachromatic mucin.
(Taylor's blue × 480.)

CHONDROBLASTOMA
Chondroblastoma is dealt with in Chapter 5 with other giant-cell lesions.

CHONDROMYXOID FIBROMA
Chondromyxoid fibroma (*Figs.* 3.32 and 3.33) is a benign tumour characterized by a proliferation of myxoid, chondroid and fibrocytoid cells arranged in lobular aggregates. The peripheral or 'growth' edge of the lobules is relatively devoid of myxoid matrix, so that the component cells are relatively closely packed there (*Fig.* 3.32). Numbers of osteoclasts also tend to aggregate along the periphery of the lobules. The more central areas of the lobules, forming the bulk of the lesion, are rich in matrix (*Fig.* 3.33) which is mainly myxoid but may be partly chondroid or chondrofibroid. The tumour is more related to chondroid neoplasms than to fibromas, and might have been better termed 'fibromyxoid chondroma'.

Cytological smears (*Fig.* 3.34) show an admixture of stellate myxoid cells, elongated fusiform fibrocytoid cells, and numbers of chondroid cells with a tendency to orange-red cytoplasm with HE. Some of the chondroid cells may have double or multiple nuclei. Viewed superficially such multinucleate cells may appear similar to those of chondrosarcomas, but the nuclei tend to be degenerate and vacuolated or dark and condensed. Scattered osteoclasts can be found in most fields. The background, in common with all chondroid tumours, stains metachromatically with Taylor's blue (*Fig.* 3.35). No alkaline phosphatase is demonstrable in the tumour cells.

CHORDOMA
Chordoma, which arises from notochordal remnants along the axial skeleton, has been dealt with in this chapter, not because it is related to cartilaginous tumours, but because on occasion it may be mistaken for chondrosarcoma. Some chordomas may contain areas with a chondroid appearance and a matrix which may be difficult to distinguish from that of chondrosarcoma. Histologically, the typical chordoma (*Fig.* 3.36) shows large pale cells which may grow in diffuse sheets or nodules but are more often arranged in cords embedded in mucinous matrix. There is some nuclear pleomorphism and giant tumour cells may be present, with a single large nucleus or with multiple nuclei, giving the tumour an ominous appearance. Mitoses are rare, but can usually be found when searched for. Glycogen is demonstrable in the cytoplasm (*Fig.* 3.37) and many cells secrete mucin (*Fig.* 3.38). The mucin may be seen in discrete vacuoles scattered throughout the cytoplasm, but tends to accumulate in a single large globule which markedly distends the cell, displacing and flattening the nucleus, producing the characteristic physaliphorous cell of 'large signet-ring' appearance. The so-called 'stromal mucin' separating the cords of tumour presumably derives from such mucus-laden cells.

Smears from a chordoma (*Figs.* 3.39–42) clearly show the constituent cells in all their different forms. A proportion of cells are devoid of intracytoplasmic mucin and, in their cytoplasmic and nuclear size and glycogen content (*Fig.* 3.40), closely resemble the cells of a low-grade chondrosarcoma. Small globules of metachromatic mucin can be found in a fair proportion of tumour cells. The physaliphorous cells (*Figs.* 3.39–42), in their huge blisters, contain a mucoid secretion (*Figs.* 3.41 and 3.42) which may be only faintly or may be moderately or quite heavily metachromatic. Scattered giant tumour cells with a single large nucleus or multiple nuclei (*Fig.* 3.39) can be seen. Mitotic figures are not frequent. Background metachromasia of varying intensity is present (*Figs.* 3.41 and 3.42). Enzyme studies are not informative in chordoma.

We consider that these cytological features are strikingly characteristic of chordoma. Metachromasia of the cytoplasm may occur in the more differentiated chondroblastic cells of chondrosarcoma, but this tends to be maximal at the periphery where it merges into the pericellular ring of matrix. Occasional globules of mucin do occur in a few cells in myxoid chondrosarcomas, but are never of the giant size noted in chordomas. Large globules of mucin may occasionally be seen in chondroblastic osteosarcoma, but the cytomorphology and cytochemistry of that condition is strikingly different from chordoma. It is sometimes said that chordoma may be mistaken for renal-cell carcinoma because of the glycogen content, but mucin production is not a feature of renal carcinomas.

References

Dahlin D.C. (1967) *Bone Tumors*, 2nd ed. Springfield, Ill., Thomas, p.147.

Gomori G. (1939) Microtechnical demonstration of phosphatase in tissue sections. *Proc. Soc. Expt. Biol. Med.* **42**, 23.

Gottschalk R.G. and Smith R.T. (1963) Chondrosarcoma of the hand: report of a case with radioactive sulphur studies and review of literature. *J. Bone Joint Surg.* **45-A**, 141.

Lichtenstein L. (1972) *Bone Tumors*, 4th ed. St Louis, Mosby, pp. 70–88, 190–214.

Lichtenstein L. and Bernstein D. (1959) Unusual benign and malignant chondroid tumors of bone. A survey of some mesenchymal cartilage tumors and malignant chondroblastic tumors, including a few multicentric ones, as well as many atypical benign chondroblastomas and chondromyxoid fibromas. *Cancer* **12**, 1142.

Lichtenstein L. and Jaffe H.L. (1943) Chondrosarcoma of bone. *Am. J. Pathol.* **19**, 553.

Remagen W., Gudat F. and Heitz P. (1976) Histochemical and electron-microscopic aspects of bone tumor diagnosis. In: Grundmann E. (ed.), *Malignant Bone Tumors*. Berlin, Springer-Verlag, p. 157.

Salzer-Kuntschik M. (1976) Cytologic and cytochemical behaviour of primary malignant bone tumors. In: Grundmann E. (ed.), *Malignant Bone Tumors*. Berlin, Springer-Verlag, p. 145.

Chapter 4

Fibrous and Fibroblastic Lesions

Non-ossifying fibroma and chondromyxoid fibroma, despite their appellation as fibromas, will not be dealt with in this chapter. Chondromyxoid fibroma has been dealt with in the chapter on cartilage tumours, because we believe it is essentially a chondroid tumour and because it is sometimes histologically confused with chondrosarcoma. Non-ossifying fibroma will be dealt with in the chapter on giant-celled lesions, because it may sometimes be mistaken for giant-cell tumour and is fundamentally a fibrohistiocytic, not a purely fibrocytic, lesion.

Fibrous and fibroblastic lesions are relatively difficult to smear and usually yield a scanty cell population. The difficulty in smearing is directly related to the amount of collagen present in the lesional tissue. Nevertheless, even well-collagenized lesions, including sclerotic fibrosarcomas, will produce enough lesional cells in their smears, provided that the smearing is performed in the manner recommended in the introductory chapter—the tissue must be crushed between the forceps and the material so expressed spread onto the slide.

FIBROUS DYSPLASIA
Fibrous dysplasia of bone is believed to be a non-neoplastic developmental anomaly which histologically presents as a fibrous lesion in which ossicles of non-lamellar fibre bone are formed in irregular islands, trabeculae and curlicues (*Fig.* 4.1). These ossicles are not rimmed by osteoblasts and strands of collagenous matrix extend directly into their substance from the surrounding fibrous tissues.

Smears from fibrous dysplasia yield a relatively sparse population of well-differentiated fibrocytic-looking cells with mature ovoid or elongated nuclei (*Fig.* 4.2), clearly much smaller than those of fibromatosis or of fibrosarcoma. Unlike the cells of fibromatosis and fibrosarcoma, which are devoid of alkaline phosphatase, the apparently fibrocytic cells of fibrous dysplasia contain this enzyme (*Figs.* 4.3 and 4.4). This fact, and their manifest capability to form fibre bone, strongly suggests that the fibrocytic-looking cells of fibrous dysplasia are in reality modified or deviant forms of osteoblasts (Changus, 1957). In this respect one might regard them as the non-neoplastic counterparts of the alkaline phosphatase containing malignant spindle-cells of fibroblastic osteosarcoma.

NON-OSSIFYING FIBROMA (*see* Chapter 5)

CHONDROMYXOID FIBROMA (*see* Chapter 3)

DESMOPLASTIC FIBROMA
This is a rare tumour of bone which histologically resembles the 'desmoid tumours'

or musculo-aponeurotic fibromatoses of the somatic soft tissues. The practical distinction between desmoplastic fibroma and well-differentiated fibrosarcoma may be difficult (Schajowicz et al., 1972). The rarity of this tumour is emphasized by the fact that relatively few well-documented cases have been reported in the literature and Dahlin has seen only 3 examples in nearly 4000 tumours of bone (Dahlin, 1967). No example has been recorded in this Registry and hence no smears are available for us to illustrate its cytology. We propose, therefore, to demonstrate instead the cytology of musculo-aponeurotic fibromatosis which is essentially similar in its structure to desmoplastic fibroma of bone.

MUSCULO-APONEUROTIC FIBROMATOSIS

The so-called 'extra-abdominal desmoid' is a locally aggressive fibroblastic proliferation which intimately infiltrates the adjoining tissues, is difficult to eradicate by local excision, has a notorious tendency to repeated recurrence, and may, on occasion, be difficult to differentiate histologically from well-differentiated fibrosarcoma.

The example to be illustrated here occurred between the os calcis and the tendo Achilles, infiltrated the tissues around the tendons, nerves and blood vessels bordering the ankle, proved impossible to remove adequately, recurred on five occasions, extended into the adjoining bones (*Fig.* 4.5), and finally forced amputation of the leg many years after its first presentation. A similar succession of events has been observed in this Registry with musculo-aponeurotic fibromatosis at several other sites, including the forearm and the upper thigh.

Histologically, musculo-aponeurotic fibromatosis shows a florid fibroblastic proliferation (*Fig.* 4.6), without any sharp line of demarcation from the host tissues, intimately and irregularly infiltrating the latter. The lesion does not show any pleomorphism, tends to produce abundant collagenous matrix, and mitoses are relatively scanty.

Cytological smears from fibromatosis (*Fig.* 4.7) show active fibroblastic cells, predominantly fusiform, with ovoid or elongated nuclei. There is a relative uniformity in the size and appearance of the fibroblasts and their nuclei, and mitoses are infrequent. The nuclear size in musculo-aponeurotic fibromatosis is demonstrably larger than in fibrous dysplasia, but smaller than in fibrosarcoma (*see* outline drawings on p. 80).

Alkaline phosphatase is absent from the lesional cells, as in fibrosarcoma.

FIBROSARCOMA OF BONE

Fibrosarcoma of bone has been defined as a primary malignant fibroblastic tumour that, upon thorough histological sampling, fails to exhibit any tendency to form tumour osteoid and bone, either in its local growth or in its metastases (Lichtenstein, 1972). The operative and essential word in this definition must be *fibroblastic*, but unfortunately with routine histological criteria it is impossible to decide whether any given spindle-cell is fibroblastic, since osteosarcoma cells can also be spindle-shaped as in the so-called 'fibroblastic' osteosarcoma. Any spindle-cell sarcoma must be shown to be devoid of alkaline phosphatase before it can be accepted as a fibrosarcoma.

As has already been stressed in the chapter on osteoblastic lesions, a number of fibroblastic osteosarcomas may not produce tumour osteoid in the sampled tissue, and by the usual histological definition must be diagnosed as fibrosarcoma. There is a group of presumed fibrosarcomas of bone which are highly malignant

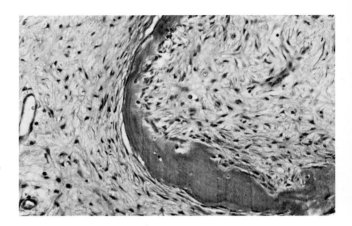

Fig. 4.1. **Fibrous dysplasia.**
Typical histology, with a
curlicue of fibre bone in a
loose fibro-cellular stroma.
(HE × 192.)

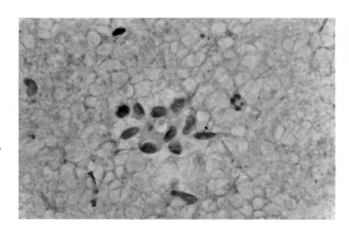

Fig. 4.2. **Fibrous dysplasia.**
Same case as in *Fig.* 4.1.
Smear showing group of
lesional cells with ovoid and
elongated nuclei;
morphologically fibrocytic.
(HE × 480.)

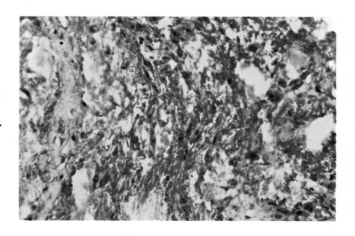

Fig. 4.3. **Fibrous dysplasia.**
Another case. Cryostat
section showing abundance
of alkaline phosphatase in
the 'fibrocytes', which are
presumably modified or
metamorphic osteoblasts.
(Alkaline phosphatase
preparation × 192.)

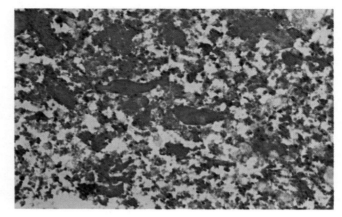

Fig. 4.4. **Fibrous dysplasia.** Same case as in *Fig.* 4.3. Smear showing two fusiform cells rich in alkaline phosphatase. Extensive background staining is present, due to release of enzyme from ruptured cells. (Alkaline phosphatase preparation × 480.)

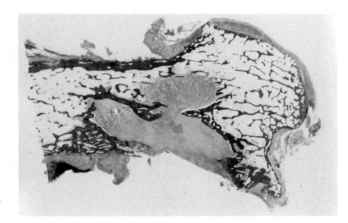

Fig. 4.5. **Musculo-aponeurotic fibromatosis.** Mounted section of distal fibula showing invasion of the bone. The distal tibia was similarly invaded. (Blue trichrome × 2·4.)

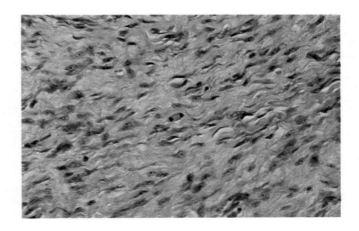

Fig. 4.6. **Musculo-aponeurotic fibromatosis.** Typical fibroblastic proliferation in a collagenous matrix. A mitosis is shown in this field, but these are not frequent. Desmoplastic fibroma of bone presents a similar pattern. (HE × 192.)

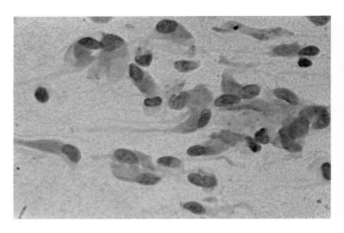

Fig. 4.7. **Musculo-aponeurotic fibromatosis.** Same case as in *Figs.* 4.5 and 4.6. Smear showing fusiform cells with ovoid and elongated nuclei. Compare nuclear size with fibrous dysplasia (*Fig.* 4.2) and low-grade fibrosarcoma (*Fig.* 4.9). (HE × 480.)

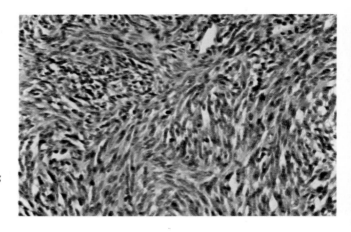

Fig. 4.8. **Well-differentiated fibrosarcoma.** Histology of tumour showing fusiform cells arranged in intersecting bands. No significant nuclear pleomorphism. (HE × 192.)

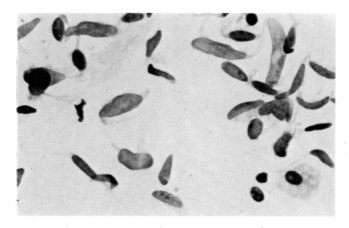

Fig. 4.9. **Well-differentiated fibrosarcoma.** Same case as in *Fig.* 4.8. Smear showing tumour cells with elongated nuclei and scanty cytoplasm; numbers of cells with smaller nuclei also present. (Giemsa × 480.)

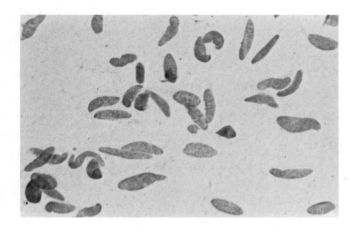

Fig. 4.10. **Well-differentiated fibrosarcoma.** Same case as in *Figs.* 4.8 and 4.9. No alkaline phosphatase is demonstrable in the tumour cells. (Alkaline phosphatase preparation × 480.)

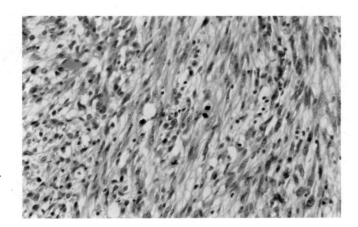

Fig. 4.11. **Poorly-differentiated fibrosarcoma.** Histology of tumour, showing a spindle-cell tumour with frequent mitoses. (HE × 192.)

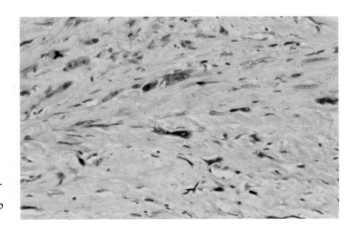

Fig. 4.12. **Poorly-differentiated fibrosarcoma.** Same case as in *Fig.* 4.11. Densely collagenized part of tumour. Tumour cells rather scanty; a tripolar mitosis is seen (top left). (HE × 192.)

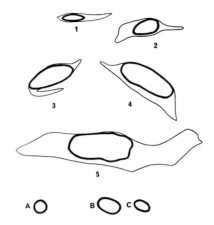

Line drawings of representative cells from fibrous dysplasia, fibromatosis and fibrosarcoma. Osteoclast and small lymphocyte nuclei are also given for comparison.

These and all other line drawings in this volume have been drawn at the same magnification.
1. Fibrous dysplasia (cell from *Fig.* 4.2).
2. Fibromatosis (cell from *Fig.* 4.7).
3. Low-grade fibrosarcoma (cell from *Fig.* 4.9).
4. High-grade fibrosarcoma (cell from *Fig.* 4.13).
5. High-grade fibrosarcoma (cell from *Fig.* 4.15).
A. Nucleus of small lymphocyte.
B. Nucleus of juvenile osteoclast.
C. Nucleus of mature osteoclast.

The nucleus in fibrous dysplasia conforms in size to that of a quiescent fibrocyte, and is much smaller than the nucleus of an active fibroblast from fibromatosis. The nuclear size in fibromatosis approximates to that of a juvenile osteoclast. The nuclei in fibrosarcoma are obviously much larger than those in fibromatosis.

neoplasms which, by virtue of their rapid and aggressive growth, their ominous cytology, and their tendency to early pulmonary metastasis, behave not unlike osteogenic sarcomas (Lichtenstein, 1972). Since histochemistry or cytochemistry has not usually been performed on such tumours, it cannot be said that they are *not* fibroblastic osteosarcomas. We have seen a number of spindle-cell sarcomas without osteoid which proved to be fibroblastic osteosarcomas on histochemical or cytochemical study. There have also been examples of osteoblastic or mixed osteosarcomas of which the metastases were spindle-celled and devoid of osteoid, but nevertheless histochemically and cytochemically osteosarcomatous, and not fibrosarcomatous.

We would therefore prefer to define fibrosarcoma of bone as 'a primary malignant *fibroblastic* tumour' or as 'a primary spindle-cell sarcoma whose cells do not contain alkaline phosphatase'.

The grading of fibrosarcomas is not always easy. Well-differentiated and anaplastic types can be readily differentiated from one another, but examples of moderately-differentiated fibrosarcoma may be difficult to separate from well-differentiated tumours at one end of their spectrum and from poorly-differentiated ones at the other. We therefore prefer to deal with two broad groups, the relatively well-differentiated and the relatively poorly-differentiated fibrosarcomas.

Well-differentiated fibrosarcoma

The example illustrated (*Figs.* 4.8–10) occurred in the tibia of a 20-year-old man, repeatedly recurred after local resection and was eventually eradicated by amputation 6 years after first presentation. Histologically, the tumour is composed of fairly uniform densely-packed spindle-shaped cells arranged in broad interlacing bundles (*Fig.* 4.8), producing orientated reticulin fibres with relatively scanty collagen. Tumour giant-cells are absent. Mitoses are present but relatively scanty and of normal type.

Cytologically (*Fig.* 4.9) the tumour cells are fusiform with elongated nuclei, without any of the pleomorphism evident in poorly-differentiated fibrosarcomas. No alkaline phosphatase (*Fig.* 4.10) is demonstrable in the tumour cells.

The difficulty in distinguishing well-differentiated fibrosarcoma from desmo-plastic fibroma has already been referred to; the nuclear size in cytological smears might well be a guide in differentiating these from one another.

Poorly-differentiated fibrosarcoma

Poorly-differentiated fibrosarcomas (*Figs.* 4.11, 4.12) show spindle-celled areas but a variable proportion of the tumour cells are of irregular shape and size, tumour giant-cells with large or multiple nuclei occur, mitoses are frequent and may be abnormal in type. A variable degree of collagen production may occur, and strands of coarse collagen may undergo hyalinization in which case it is important not to mistake them for osteoidal matrix.

Cytologically, poorly-differentiated fibrosarcomas display fusiform cells with elongated or ovoid nuclei (*Fig.* 4.13), but cells with rounded, polyhedral or stellate shapes are also seen (*Fig.* 4.14), together with giant tumour cells with huge or multiple nuclei. Mitoses, including abnormal ones, can be found (*Fig.* 4.16). No alkaline phosphatase is demonstrable in the tumour cells (*Figs.* 4.15 and 4.16) and it is this feature which ultimately distinguishes fibrosarcoma from fibroblastic osteosarcoma.

The diagnostic confusion between fibrosarcoma and fibroblastic osteosarcoma, inevitable when the diagnosis is based simply on routine histological stains, and between fibrosarcoma and malignant fibrous histiocytoma (*see* Chapter 10), may account for the divergence of opinion concerning the prognosis of fibrosarcoma of bone. According to some writers (McLeod et al., 1957; Gilmer and MacEwen, 1958; Dahlin and Ivins, 1969), the 5-year survival rate in fibrosarcoma is not nearly so good as that of somatic soft-tissue fibrosarcoma, but better than that of osteosarcoma. Others (Larsson et al., 1976) found the prognosis to be much worse than in osteosarcoma. In a study by Jeffree and Price (1976), the prognosis of fibrosarcoma differed very little from that of osteosarcoma, *for similar age groups*, but most of their cases were diagnosed before histochemical or cytochemical studies were available. It is highly probable that all these series must have included a certain number of spindle-cell osteosarcomas and malignant fibrous histiocy-tomas, and their results must be viewed with this probability in mind.

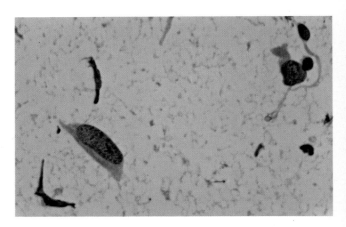

Fig. 4.13. **Poorly-differentiated fibrosarcoma.** Same case as in *Figs.* 4.11, 4.12. Smear showing two large tumour cells: one with elongated nucleus (below left), one with rounded nucleus (top right). (HE × 480.)

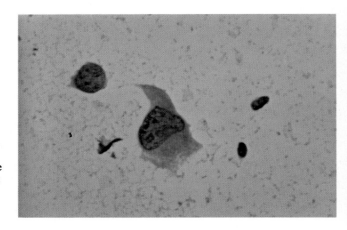

Fig. 4.14. **Poorly-differentiated fibrosarcoma.** Same case as in *Figs.* 4.11–13. Giant tumour cell with single large nucleus. Another malignant cell shows a round nucleus and scanty cytoplasm. (HE × 480.)

Fig. 4.15. **Poorly-differentiated fibrosarcoma.** Another case. Smear showing several tumour cells, including a large fusiform cell with elongated hyperchromatic nucleus. No alkaline phosphatase is present in the tumour cells. Because no enzyme staining is demonstrable, the nucleus is clearly visible. (Alkaline phosphatase preparation × 480.)

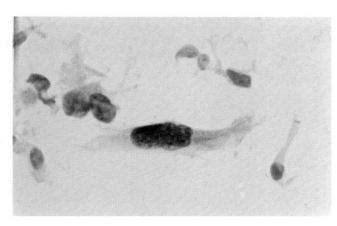

Fig. 4.16. **Poorly-differentiated fibrosarcoma.** Another case. Many of the tumour cells have round or ovoid, not fusiform, nuclei. Two cells are seen in mitosis, one of them being much larger than the other cells. No alkaline phosphatase is demonstrable. (Alkaline phosphatase preparation × 480.)

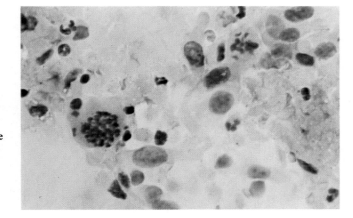

References

Changus G.W. (1957) Osteoblastic hyperplasia of bone: histochemical appraisal of fibrous dysplasia of bone. *Cancer 10*, 1157.

Dahlin D.C. (1967) *Bone Tumors*, 2nd ed. Springfield, Ill., Thomas, p. 219.

Dahlin D.C. and Ivins J.C. (1969) Fibrosarcoma of bone: a study of 114 cases. *Cancer 23*, 35.

Gilmer W.S. and MacEwen G.D. (1958) Central (medullary) fibrosarcoma of bone. *J. Bone Joint Surg. 40-A*, 121.

Jeffree G.M. and Price C.H.G. (1976) Metastatic spread of fibrosarcoma of bone: a report on 49 cases, and a comparison with osteosarcoma. *J. Bone Joint Surg. 58-B*, 418.

Larrson S.-E., Lorentzon R. and Boquist L. (1976) Fibrosarcoma of bone: a demographic, clinical and histopathological study of all cases recorded in the Swedish Cancer Registry from 1958 to 1968. *J. Bone Joint Surg. 58-B*, 412.

Lichtenstein L. (1972) *Bone Tumors*, 4th ed. St Louis, Mosby, pp. 244, 250.

McLeod J.J., Dahlin D.C. and Ivins J.C. (1957) Fibrosarcoma of bone. *Am. J. Surg. 94*, 431.

Schajowicz F., Ackerman L.V. and Sissons H.A. (1972) *Histological Typing of Bone Tumours*. Geneva, WHO, p. 42.

Chapter 5

Giant-cell-containing Lesions

Apart from giant-cell tumour of bone, a wide variety of intra-osseous lesions may contain abundant osteoclasts, either throughout the entire lesion or in selected samples. With some of these lesions, on occasions, a fallacious diagnosis of giant-cell tumour may be made, particularly if limited material is examined and the histology is viewed out of context with the clinical and radiological features.

Aneurysmal bone cyst will be discussed in Chapter 9, with cystic lesions of bone. Chondromyxoid fibroma has been discussed with the cartilage tumours (Chapter 3). Osteoclast-rich osteosarcoma has been discussed with the other types of osteosarcoma (Chapter 2). We have chosen to deal with non-ossifying fibroma and benign chondroblastoma in this Chapter, rather than with fibrous and chondroid tumours respectively, in order to stress some of the histological and cytological resemblances they have to giant-cell tumour of bone.

NON-OSSIFYING FIBROMA

Two relatively common benign lesions of bone, fibrous cortical defect and metaphysial fibrous defect, present identical histological appearances—that of non-ossifying fibroma (*Figs.* 5.1–4). This is a fibro-histiocytic, rather than a purely fibrocytic, proliferation showing oval or fusiform stromal cells arranged in interlacing bundles or whorls, often with a storiform pattern (*Fig.* 5.1), accompanied by variable numbers of osteoclasts. The osteoclastic population may be relatively scanty but at times is quite abundant (*Fig.* 5.2.), in which case the lesion may resemble osteoclastoma and, if the clinical and radiological features are disregarded, may be misdiagnosed as such. The stromal cells tend to undergo foam-cell change, and parts of the lesion may become extensively xanthomatous (*Fig.* 5.3); occasional examples may be predominantly xanthomatous and may then be labelled as 'xanthoma', 'fibro-xanthoma' or 'xantho-granuloma'. Such foam-cell change is entirely non-specific and may be seen in many other intra-osseous lesions, including giant-cell tumour and histiocytosis X. Haemosiderin also tends to accumulate within the stromal cells, with or without known antecedent trauma. Osteoidal matrix may be found in non-ossifying fibroma, sometimes reactive to trauma, sometimes as a metaplastic process intrinsic to the lesion (*Fig.* 5.4). Mitoses are rare, but they do occur.

Smears from non-ossifying fibroma (*Figs.* 5.5 and 5.6) show an admixture of ovoid and fusiform stromal cells with elongated nuclei as well as rounded histiocytic-type cells with round or oval nuclei. Osteoclasts are usually present, and may be abundant or sparse depending on their prevalence in the sampled lesion. Similarly, the presence and numbers of lipid-laden foam cells (*Figs.* 5.6 and 5.7) and haemosiderin-containing cells (*Fig.* 5.8) will depend on their proportions in

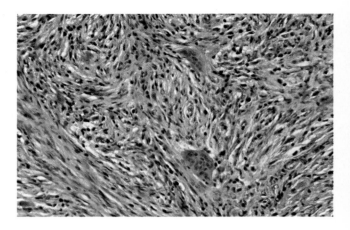

Fig. 5.1. **Non-ossifying fibroma.** Typical storiform pattern of fusiform 'fibrocytic' cells, with several osteoclasts. Rounded of ovoid mononuclear cells are present in such areas but these cannot be identified with any certainty in histological sections, because the fusiform cells sectioned transversely would look much the same. (HE × 192.)

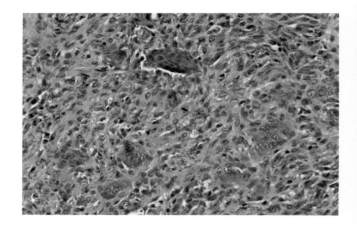

Fig. 5.2. **Non-ossifying fibroma.** Another case. Example which may be easily mistaken for a giant-cell tumour, because of presence of abundant osteoclasts. Other fields showed typical storiform pattern, as in *Fig.* 5.1 above. Clinically and radiologically, the lesion fully conformed to metaphysial fibrous defect, *not* to giant-cell tumour. (HE × 192.)

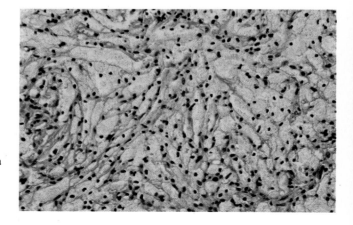

Fig. 5.3. **Non-ossifying fibroma.** Another case. Area in which the lesional cells have undergone extensive foam-cell change. (HE × 192.)

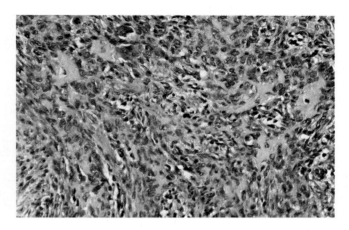

Fig. 5.4. **Non-ossifying fibroma.** Another case. Field showing patchy osteoidal metaplasia, intrinsic to the lesion. Such intrinsic osteoid formation may also be seen in giant-cell tumours. Examples such as this tend to be relatively rich in alkaline phosphatase. (HE × 192.)

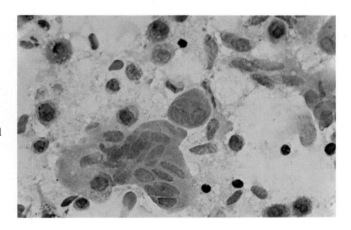

Fig. 5.5. **Non-ossifying fibroma.** Same case as in *Fig.* 5.1. Typical cytological field containing two osteoclasts. The stromal cells include fusiform cells with elongated nuclei as well as rounded histiocytic cells. A number of these have vacuolated eosinophilic cytoplasm, due to active phagocytosis of lipid and blood pigment. (HE × 480.)

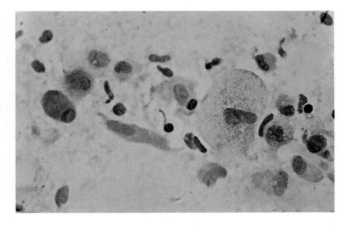

Fig. 5.6. **Non-ossifying fibroma.** Same case as in *Figs.* 5.1 and 5.5. Field from smear showing a large bloated foam cell and several smaller not fully developed foam cells. Histiocytes with blood pigment are also present, together with a fusiform 'fibrocytic' cell and a typical normal osteoblast with its racket-shape and eccentric nucleus (on left). (HE × 480.)

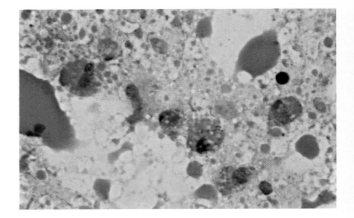

Fig. 5.7. **Non-ossifying fibroma.** Same case as in Fig. 5.3. Smear showing several lipid-containing foam cells. Many of these cells rupture, spreading amorphous extracellular lipid on the slide. (Oil Red O × 480.)

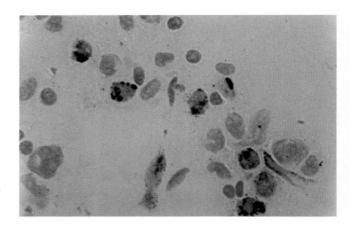

Fig. 5.8. **Non-ossifying fibroma.** Same case as in Figs. 5.1, 5.5 and 5.6. Smear showing haemosiderin-laden cells. Perl's positive material is present in both rounded and fusiform cells. (Perl's × 480.)

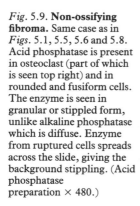

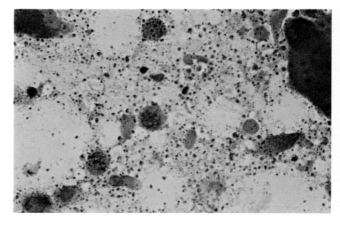

Fig. 5.9. **Non-ossifying fibroma.** Same case as in Figs. 5.1, 5.5, 5.6 and 5.8. Acid phosphatase is present in osteoclast (part of which is seen top right) and in rounded and fusiform cells. The enzyme is seen in granular or stippled form, unlike alkaline phosphatase which is diffuse. Enzyme from ruptured cells spreads across the slide, giving the background stippling. (Acid phosphatase preparation × 480.)

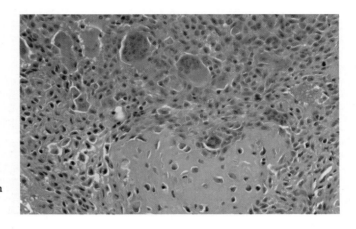

Fig. 5.10. **Benign chondroblastoma.** Histological field showing (top half) an admixture of osteoclasts and juvenile or partly matured chondroblasts; the latter may be mistaken for the stromal cells of a giant-cell tumour. A well-defined nodule of cartilage is seen in bottom half of field. (HE × 192.)

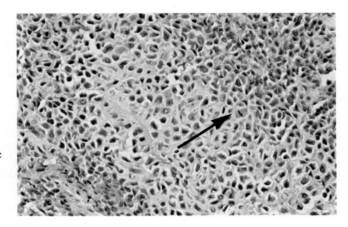

Fig. 5.11. **Benign chondroblastoma.** Another case. Typical histological field showing chondroblastic maturation with chondroid matrix, but without mature cartilage. Note cell in mitosis (arrowed). (HE × 192.)

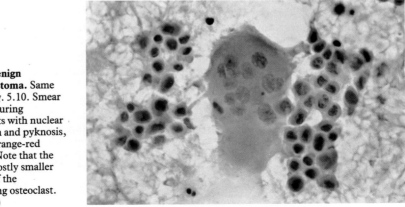

Fig. 5.12. **Benign chondroblastoma.** Same case as in *Fig*. 5.10. Smear showing maturing chondroblasts with nuclear condensation and pyknosis, and bright orange-red cytoplasm. Note that the nuclei are mostly smaller than those of the accompanying osteoclast. (HE × 480.)

the sampled lesion. Mitoses, if present, are quite infrequent. Osteoblasts may be found (*Fig.* 5.6), depending on the presence and extent of osteoidal tissue in the sample smeared. Any alkaline phosphatase in the smears is usually confined to osteoblasts and endothelial cells; but in occasional cases, a certain amount of alkaline phosphatase may be present in some of the lesional cells. Acid phosphatase is present in the osteoclasts and in many of the stromal cells (*Fig.* 5.9) and reinforces the view that the latter are fundamentally histiocytic. Background metachromasia is absent.

The cytology of non-ossifying fibroma is frequently characteristic enough to permit a confident diagnosis, certainly in correlation with the clinical and radiological data. Smears with abundant osteoclasts may resemble those of giant-cell tumour, but mitoses are rare in non-ossifying fibroma whilst they are easy to find in giant-cell tumour. Non-ossifying fibromas which have undergone extensive foam-cell change may be cytologically difficult to differentiate from other lesions which have undergone similar xanthomatous change, but such extreme instances are exceptional. The lesional tissue in the lining of a simple bone cyst contains variable admixtures of fusiform and rounded cells as well as some osteoclasts, and its smears may occasionally show a cell population similar to that seen in non-ossifying fibroma; in non-ossifying fibroma, however, the smear contains abundant cells whereas the smear of a simple bone cyst is extremely sparse.

The cytology of non-ossifying fibroma indicates that it is really a fibro-histiocytic lesion, not a true fibrous one. This suggestion has already been made by Huvos (1976) in his account of malignant fibrous histiocytoma of bone. He pointed out that, since there are many examples of benign fibrous histiocytomas in soft tissues, benign counterparts of malignant fibrous histiocytoma are also a real possibility in bone, and that 'such lesions as non-ossifying fibroma and fibro-xanthoma could be regarded as benign tumours of fibrous histiocytic origin'. Despite its time-honoured appellation as a 'fibroma', non-ossifying fibroma differs from fibrous dysplasia, which is a metamorphic osteoblastic lesion (Changus, 1957) with fusiform alkaline phosphatase-positive cells, and from desmoplastic fibroma of which the cells are genuinely fibroblastic, and, on the analogy of musculo-aponeurotic fibromatosis which it closely resembles, without acid or alkaline phosphatase.

BENIGN CHONDROBLASTOMA

Benign chondroblastoma is characterized by a proliferation of non-malignant chondroblasts which show varying degrees of maturation and differentiation, varying from tumour to tumour, and in various parts of the same tumour. The less mature chondroblasts may closely resemble the stromal cells of a giant-cell tumour and are often accompanied by an abundance of osteoclasts, so that biopsies from such areas, or from tumours predominantly of such structure (*Fig.* 5.10), may resemble osteoclastoma and, by the inexpert, be mistaken for it. The more mature chondroblasts (*Fig.* 5.11) have condensed nuclei and lie in a chondroid matrix. In places, often in circumscribed islands, fully mature cartilage (*Fig.* 5.10) may form and may undergo degenerative change, necrosis and calcification.

Smears from benign chondroblastoma (*Figs.* 5.12–16) show an admixture of osteoclasts and chondroblasts in various stages of development and maturation. Patches of background metachromasia may be seen (*Fig.* 5.15). The nuclei of the younger, less mature cells (*Fig.* 5.13) are often larger than osteoclastic nuclei, appear ovoid or spherical, and have delicate stippled chromatin network; their cytoplasm is pale and lightly eosinophilic. The more mature cells (*Figs.* 5.12 and 5.14) undergo progressive condensation of their nuclei which eventually become shrunken, distorted or crenellated; their cytoplasm becomes increasingly eosinophilic and orange-red with Eosin. Mitoses can be found with greater ease than in ossifying fibroma, but are never frequent. Acid phosphatase is found in the osteoclasts and sometimes in a proportion of the stromal cells, but is not seen in the differentiated chondroblastic cells. Glycogen is present in some of the more mature chondroblastic cells (*Fig.* 5.16).

A specific feature helps differentiate smears of osteoclast-rich benign chondroblastoma from giant-cell tumour—metachromasia of the background with Taylor's blue is present in chondroblastoma but not in giant-cell tumour.

ANEURYSMAL BONE CYST (*see* Chapter 9)

CHONDROMYXOID FIBROMA (*see* Chapter 3)

OSTEOCLAST-RICH OSTEOSARCOMA (*see* Chapter 2)

'BROWN TUMOUR' OF HYPERPARATHYROIDISM

The 'brown tumour' of hyperparathyroidism may be difficult to distinguish from giant-cell tumour and misdiagnoses may occur if a given lesion is assessed without reference to the clinical, radiological and biochemical data, or to the histology of the osseous tissue beyond the lesion. No example of this lesion has come to be smeared in this laboratory, but a number of cases have been examined histochemically in which acid phosphatase has been demonstrable in the osteoclasts and in some of the stromal cells. We strongly suspect that smears from this condition might prove difficult to distinguish from those of conventional giant-cell tumours.

GIANT-CELL TUMOUR OF BONE (OSTEOCLASTOMA)

Giant-cell tumour of bone is a relatively uncommon tumour; about 1 case is seen for every 4 cases of osteosarcoma. For this reason, relatively few cases have been studied here cytologically, mainly in the last few years, and all have been conventional giant-cell tumours. Frankly sarcomatous giant-cell tumours are very rare and usually arise after irradiation of a conventional giant-cell tumour; no recent example has been recorded in this Registry.

Conventional giant-cell tumour has been subject to much controversy concerning its grading (Jaffe et al., 1940). Lichtenstein (1972) maintains that grading is of value in the assessment of giant-cell tumours of bone, in that an aggressive clinical course is more likely in Grade II tumours than in Grade I. Others (Williams et al., 1954; Schajowicz, 1961; Campbell and Bonfiglio, 1973) have felt that grading of conventional giant-cell tumours has little to offer in their assessment. We confess we have found histological grading a difficult exercise and open to considerable subjective bias.

Giant-cell tumour (*Figs.* 5.17, 5.19, 5.21, 5.24) histologically shows a variable admixture of osteoclast-type multinucleate giant cells and 'stromal' cells which may be rounded, ovoid or fusiform. Cells intermediate between the typical giant cells and the mononuclear stromal cells may be found, with 2–4 nuclei. By and large, the giant cells are quite frequent and prominent, but predominantly stromal-celled areas may occur in which they may be scanty or absent. Parts of the tumour may be extensively spindle-celled and, in their structure, closely resemble non-ossifying

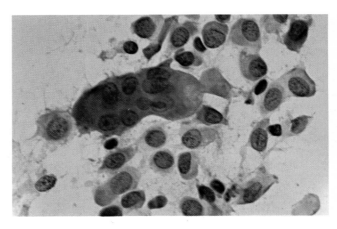

Fig. 5.13. **Benign chondroblastoma.** Same case as in *Fig.* 5.11. Smear showing juvenile chondroblasts. Most of the cells have large nuclei with fine stippled chromatin and pale cytoplasm. Nuclei tend to be larger than those of the osteoclast present in the field. (HE × 480.)

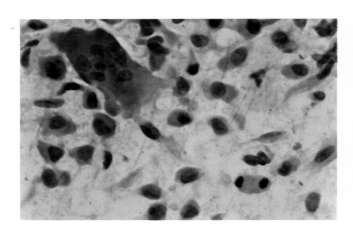

Fig. 5.14. **Benign chondroblastoma.** Same case as in *Figs.* 5.11 and 5.13. Smear showing rather less immature cells than in *Fig.* 5.13. Note cell in mitosis; these are relatively rare in benign chondroblastoma. (HE × 480.)

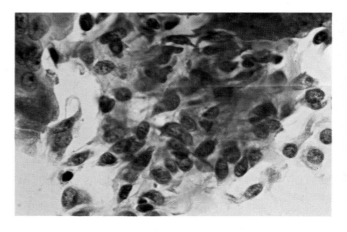

Fig. 5.15. **Benign chondroblastoma.** Same case as in *Figs.* 5.11, 5.13 and 5.14. Cluster of lesional cells with metachromasia of the background; the latter is a feature of all chondroid tumours. (Taylor's blue × 480.)

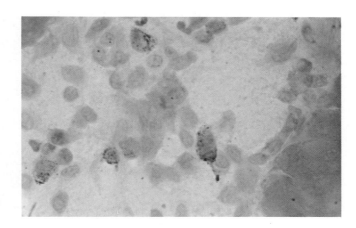

Fig. 5.16. **Benign chondroblastoma.** Same case as in *Figs.* 5.11, 5.13–15. Glycogen is present in some of the chondroblastic cells. (PAS × 480.)

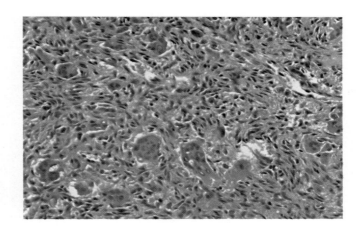

Fig. 5.17. **Giant-cell tumour.** Case 1. Histology from area showing predominantly spindle-celled stromal component with scattered osteoclasts. (HE × 192.)

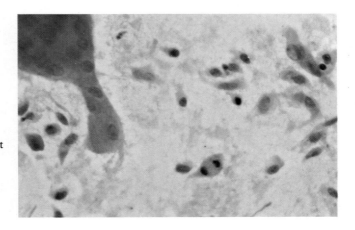

Fig. 5.18. **Giant-cell tumour.** Case 1. Smear showing part of an osteoclast and stromal cells, mostly fusiform, one in mitosis. Note that the nuclei of the stromal cells in this case are smaller than those of the osteoclast. (HE × 480.)

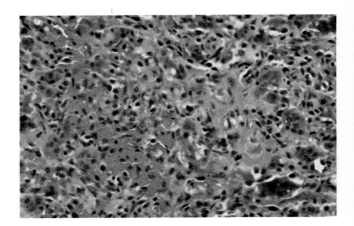

Fig. 5.19. **Giant-cell tumour.** Case 2. Histology from area with relatively scanty osteoclasts. (HE × 192.)

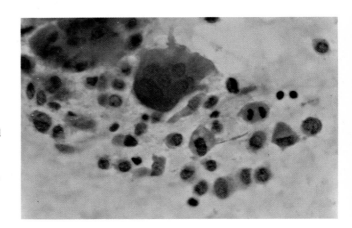

Fig. 5.20. **Giant-cell tumour.** Case 2. Smear showing two osteoclasts and stromal cells, mostly ovoid or rounded, one in mitosis. Nuclear size approximately the same as in osteoclasts or smaller. Occasional binucleate cells are present. (HE × 480.)

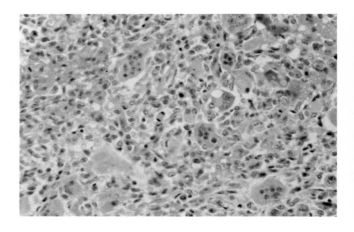

Fig. 5.21. **Giant-cell tumour.** Case 3. Histologically a conventional giant-cell tumour with rather prominent stromal cells. Several mitoses are present in this field. (HE × 192.)

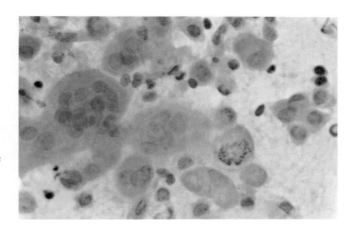

Fig. 5.22. **Giant-cell tumour.** Case 3. Smear showing osteoclasts and stromal cells. Several osteoclasts have relatively few nuclei. Two binucleate cells are seen with nuclei larger than those of the large osteoclast. A large cell in mitosis is also seen. Other stromal cells are smaller, some contain blood pigment. (HE × 480.)

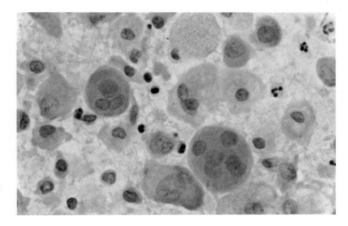

Fig. 5.23. **Giant-cell tumour.** Case 3. Smear showing osteoclasts and stromal cells. The osteoclasts have relatively few nuclei. Several stromal cells have large open nuclei, larger than those of the osteoclasts. Numerous mature stromal cells with small condensed nuclei are actively phagocytic and have abundant foamy cytoplasm. (HE × 480.)

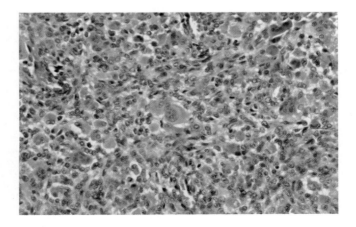

Fig. 5.24. **Giant-cell tumour.** Case 4. Histology of area showing abundant stromal cells, many binucleate, some with exceptionally large nuclei. (HE × 192.)

fibroma. Osteoid matrix may be found sometimes as an intrinsic metaplastic component of the tumour, and may rarely be extensive enough to create diagnostic difficulties by simulating osteoblastoma. Haemorrhages and haemosiderin deposition may occur. Focal foam-cell change may be found, much as in non-ossifying fibroma but as a rule less frequently and less extensively. Normal mitoses are usually found in all examples of conventional giant-cell tumour and may be quite frequent.

The representative histology and the corresponding cytology will be presented from 4 cases, giving the range of spectrum in conventional giant-cell tumour. It will be noted that the cytological smears from these cases provide a closely faithful representation of their make-up as observed in the histological sections. The relative paucity of the tumours smeared and the brevity of the follow-up period make it impossible for us to offer any opinion concerning the prognostic significance, if any, of the cytological variations observed.

Case 1. The tumour, in the left 4th metacarpal of a 26-year-old man, histologically shows a conventional pattern with abundant giant cells, in parts with fusiform fibrous-looking stromal cells (*Fig.* 5.17) having rather small nuclei, presumed to be a Grade I tumour. Mitoses are present but are less frequent than in Cases 3 and 4.

Smears (*Fig.* 5.18) illustrate that most of the stromal cells are small, ovoid or fusiform, and their nuclei are mostly smaller than those of the osteoclasts, with considerable condensation and pyknosis. Mitoses can be found fairly easily.

Case 2. A giant-cell tumour in the distal femur of a 47-year-old man (*Fig.* 5.19). Cytologically (*Fig.* 5.20), the stromal cells are again relatively small, with small round or ovoid nuclei. Occasional binucleate cells and fair numbers of mitoses are present. The degree of nuclear condensation is less marked than in Case 1.

Case 3. A giant-cell tumour in the proximal tibia of a 19-year-old woman, presenting after a pathological fracture. Histologically (*Fig.* 5.21) the stromal cells are prominent and in many fields predominant. Cytologically (*Figs.* 5.22 and 5.23) numbers of cells with exceptionally large nuclei are present, including some cells with two to four nuclei, and mitoses can be found in such intermediate-size cells. Many of the more mature cells have become bloated, with a foamy cytoplasm, and some contain blood pigment, clearly a phagocytic response to the pathological fracture. We suspect that this reactive modification may also have involved the less mature stromal cells which, like normal juvenile histiocytes, might have undergone nuclear enlargement, rendering the grading of this tumour difficult.

Case 4. This was a Grade II+ giant-cell tumour in the distal femur of a 21-year-old woman, referred to us very recently. Histologically, parts of the tumour present an average giant-celled pattern. In others (*Fig.* 5.24) giant-cells are sparse, mitoses frequent, and stromal cells with exceptionally large nuclei are present; binucleate stromal cells can be found with relative ease. Other features unrelated to grading, in that they may be found in any giant-cell tumour, include focal foam-cell change (*Fig.* 5.25) and osteoidal reaction (*Fig.* 5.26).

Cytological smears (*Figs.* 5.27–29) illustrate the less mature and to some degree more pleomorphic nature of the stromal cells. They all have relatively large nuclei with sharp finely stippled chromatin, mitoses are frequent, and binucleate forms relatively common. There is an appreciable degree of nuclear pleomorphism and occasional cells with exceptionally large, rather hyperchromatic nuclei are present. An occasional unusually large cell, probably an intermediate or small giant cell, is seen in mitosis (*Fig.* 5.29) with an obviously polyploid number of chromosomes; it may well represent an osteoclast or pro-osteoclast in mitosis.

In both its histological and cytological features, this giant-cell tumour is a fairly high-grade conventional, i.e. not sarcomatous, example and its progress is awaited with special interest. It should be noted that the high grade of this tumour is perhaps more readily appreciated in the cytological smears than in the histological sections.

Background metachromasia is absent in smears of giant-cell tumours stained with Taylor's blue. Acid phosphatase is present in the osteoclasts and to a variable but appreciable extent in the stromal cells (*Fig.* 5.30). In some cases, neutral phosphatase may also be present in these cells. It is important to bear this in mind, because some methods for the demonstration of alkaline phosphatase also demonstrate neutral phosphatase, and the latter may then erroneously be assumed to be alkaline phosphatase. In any case where alkaline phosphatase is unexpectedly or paradoxically demonstrable in any smear, special techniques should be used to prove that the enzyme in question is neutral, not alkaline, phosphatase.

We have already mentioned that the cytology of non-ossifying fibroma is that of a benign fibro-histiocytic lesion. Giant-cell tumour is also seen as a predominantly histiocytic lesion and might be considered essentially to be a form of histiocytoma. It should be remembered that osteoclasts and their mononuclear precursors are the specialized phagocytic cells of bone which normally ingest bone, but when the occasion arises they will also phagocytose other material, including blood pigment and lipids.

The cytological differentiation of giant-cell tumour from various other giant-celled lesions is briefly recapitulated below, although it will have been referred to in the accounts of those particular lesions.

1. *Non-ossifying fibroma.* The stromal cells of non-ossifying fibroma, like those of giant-cell tumour, tend to undergo differentiation into histiocytes and may contain acid phosphatase. Certain examples of non-ossifying fibroma may be somewhat similar to the smears of Grade I giant-cell tumours, but their mitotic activity is always low.

2. *Benign chondroblastoma.* Certain examples of this tumour may be cytomorphologically rather similar to giant-cell tumour of bone, but identifiable chondroblasts can usually be found and some background metachromasia will be present. Background metachromasia is absent in giant-cell tumour. Only relatively few 'stromal' cells in benign chondroblastoma contain acid phosphatase.

3. *Chondromyxoid fibroma.* This is unlikely ever to be confused with giant-cell tumour, even in smears which may contain abundant giant cells. The cytomorphology of the lesional cells differs significantly from the stromal cells of giant-cell tumour, background metachromasia is abundantly evident, and the tumour cells do not contain more than a trace of acid phosphatase.

4. *Giant-cell rich osteosarcoma.* This may be mistaken for a malignant giant-cell tumour, but its non-osteoclastic cellular component is demonstrably osteosarcomatous and rich in alkaline phosphatase, quite unlike the stromal cells of giant-cell tumour.

5. *'Brown tumour' of hyperparathyroidism.* Smears might well be indistinguishable from those of Grade I giant-cell tumour. Differentiation of this lesion from giant-cell tumour would depend on clinical, radiological and biochemical data, and on the histology of the bone beyond the lesional area.

6. *Aneurysmal bone cyst.* Examples containing abundant osteoclasts in the smears may require clinical, radiological and histological assessment for their differentiation from giant-cell tumour.

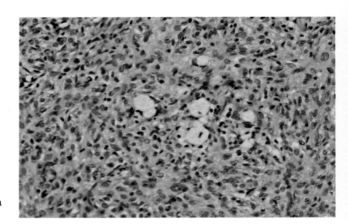

Fig. 5.25. **Giant-cell tumour.** Case 4. Histology of predominantly stromal-celled area with several foam cells. (HE × 192.)

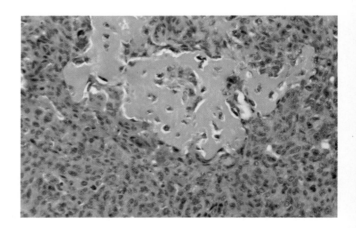

Fig. 5.26. **Giant-cell tumour.** Case 4. Osteoidal matrix in predominantly stromal-celled field. (HE × 192.)

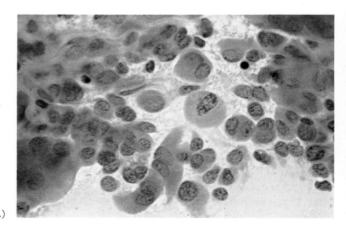

Fig. 5.27. **Giant-cell tumour.** Case 4. Representative smear. Part of an osteoclast is seen below left; part of another top right. Group of stromal cells, including many binucleate ones. Nuclei have sharp stippled chromatin. Some of the stromal cells have nuclei much larger than those of the osteoclasts. (HE × 480.)

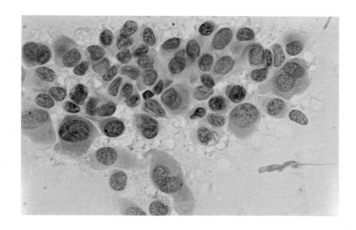

Fig. 5.28. **Giant-cell tumour.** Case 4. Smear showing a collection of stromal cells with considerable variation in nuclear size. Several cells are binucleate. Two of the mononucleate cells have unduly large nuclei. (HE × 480.)

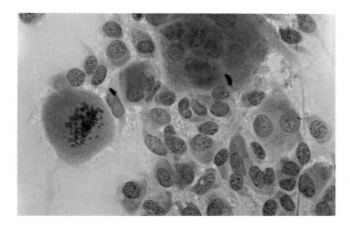

Fig. 5.29. **Giant-cell tumour.** Case 4. Smear showing typical multinucleate osteoclast above. Large binucleate cell is seen on the right; exceptionally large cell in mitosis on left. (HE × 480.)

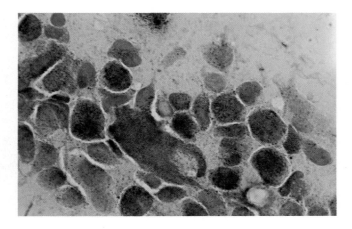

Fig. 5.30. **Giant-cell tumour.** Case 4. Smear: a small osteoclast and many stromal cells contain acid phosphatase. Many of the stromal cells in this field are binucleate. (Acid phosphatase preparation × 480.)

The nuclear size of 'stromal' cells in non-ossifying fibroma, benign chondroblastoma and giant-cell tumour of bone is demonstrated in the following black-and-white tracings, drawn at the same magnification.

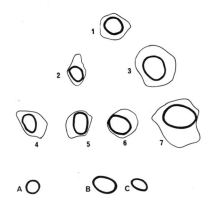

Line drawings of representative cells from non-ossifying fibroma, chondroblastoma and giant-cell tumour. Osteoclast and small lymphocyte nuclei are also given for comparison.

These and all other line drawings in this volume have been drawn at the same magnification.

1. Non-ossifying fibroma (stromal cell from *Fig.* 5.5).
2. Benign chondroblastoma (senescent chondroblast from *Fig.* 5.12).
3. Benign chondroblastoma (active or juvenile chondroblast from *Fig.* 5.13).
4. Giant-cell tumour (stromal cell from *Fig.* 5.18).
5. Giant-cell tumour (stromal cell from *Fig.* 5.20).
6. Giant-cell tumour (stromal cell from *Fig.* 5.22).
7. Giant-cell tumour (stromal cell from *Fig.* 5.28).
A. Nucleus of small lymphocyte.
B. Nucleus of juvenile osteoclast.
C. Nucleus of mature osteoclast.

Nuclear size in non-ossifying fibroma, chondroblastoma and giant-cell tumour generally approximates to that of a juvenile osteoclast but is larger than that of a mature osteoclast. Only the nucleus of a Grade II[+] giant-cell tumour (*Fig.* 5.28) is significantly larger than the nucleus of a juvenile osteoclast.

References

Campbell C.J. and Bonfiglio M. (1973) Aggressiveness and malignancy in giant-cell tumours of bone. In: Price C.H.G. and Ross F.G.M. (ed.), *Bone—Certain Aspects of Neoplasia*. London, Butterworths, p. 17.

Changus G.W. (1957) Osteoblastic hyperplasia of bone: a histochemical appraisal of fibrous dysplasia of bone. *Cancer 10*, 1157.

Huvos A.G. (1976) Primary malignant fibrous histiocytoma of bone. Clinicopathologic study of 18 patients. *N.Y. State J. Med. 76*, 552.

Jaffe H.L., Lichtenstein L. and Portis R.B. (1940) Giant cell tumor of bone: its pathologic appearance, grading, supposed variants and treatment. *Arch. Pathol. 30*, 993.

Lichtenstein L. (1972) *Bone Tumors*, 4th ed. St Louis, Mosby, pp.150–158.

Schajowicz F. (1961) Giant-cell tumors of bone (osteoclastoma). A pathological and histochemical study. *J. Bone Joint Surg. 43-A*, 1.

Williams R.R., Dahlin D.C. and Ghormley R.K. (1954) Giant-cell tumor of bone. *Cancer 7*, 764.

Chapter 6

Malignant Round-cell Tumours

The term 'malignant round-cell tumour', as used in this Registry, applies to three tumours which usually require differentiation from one another: reticulosarcoma, Ewing's tumour and metastatic neuroblastoma. Typical examples of these tumours have fairly characteristic histological and cytological features, but atypical forms do occur and may present considerable diagnostic problems.

We do not apply the term 'malignant round-cell tumour' to other tumours of diverse origin with 'round cells', but for convenience plasma-cell myeloma will also be considered in this chapter, and a brief reference will be made to alveolar rhabdomyosarcoma. We have decided not to deal with leukaemias in this volume and would refer the reader to standard haematological reference books and atlases for their cytological details.

RETICULOSARCOMA

Of malignant lymphomas, Hodgkin's disease in its various forms rarely presents clinically as a primary bone problem; osseous involvement is usually an incidental part of established disseminated disease. An occasional example has been recorded in this Registry in which Hodgkin's disease presented primarily in bone, but none has come to be smeared, so that cytological illustrations of Hodgkin's disease cannot be given in this volume. An occasional case of lymphoblastic lymphosarcoma presents primarily in bone and illustrations of such a case are given in *Figs.* 6.1 and 6.2; the admixture of lymphoblastic and lymphocytic tumour cells is clearly seen.

The variety of non-Hodgkin's malignant lymphoma usually encountered in bone tumour work is the type of reticulosarcoma designated as 'reticulum-cell sarcoma' (Parker and Jackson, 1939) or 'clasmacytoma' (Gall and Mallory, 1942). Fashions in the nomenclature of this particular tumour come and go, but we prefer to use the time-honoured term 'reticulosarcoma' because that term will be unequivocally understood by most clinicians and diagnosticians involved in the study and management of bone tumours.

Histologically, examples of reticulosarcoma are illustrated in *Figs.* 6.3–5. The tumour cells tend to be more polymorphous than in Ewing's tumour and show variations in cytoplasmic and nuclear size and shape, some nuclei being round or ovoid, others reniform or bean-shaped, indented, grooved or cleaved. The nuclei show coarsely stippled or granular chromatin, with nucleoli, or they may appear vesicular. The tumour produces abundant reticulin (*Fig.* 6.5) which may be partly pericellular and partly around small groups of cells; in parts, the latter pattern may predominate, producing an alveolar arrangement. Glycogen is absent from the

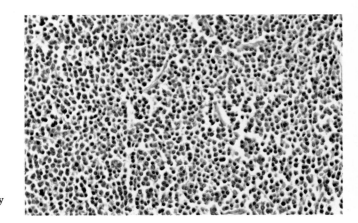

Fig. 6.1. **Lymphoblastic lymphosarcoma.** Histology of tumour. (HE × 192.)

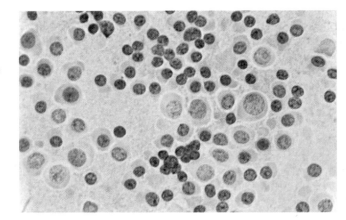

Fig. 6.2. **Lymphoblastic lymphosarcoma.** Same case as in *Fig.* 6.1. Smear showing an admixture of lymphoblasts and lymphocytes. There is some variation in nuclear size, depending on the maturity of the tumour cells, but all the nuclei are round and do not show the grooving or indentation seen in reticulosarcoma. (HE × 480.) .

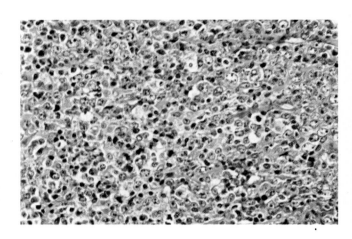

Fig. 6.3. **Reticulosarcoma.** Typical histological pattern with variations in cell and nuclear size. (HE × 192.)

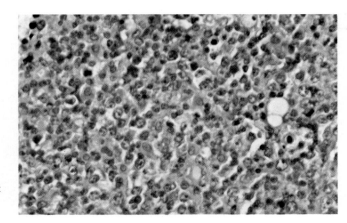

Fig. 6.4. **Reticulosarcoma.** Same case as in *Fig.* 6.3. A number of cells show abundant cytoplasm containing diastase-resistant PAS-positive material. (PAS-diastase × 192.)

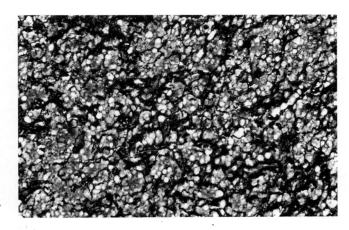

Fig. 6.5. **Reticulosarcoma.** Another case. Brisk reticulin stroma, with some tendency to parcelling around small groups of cells. (Reticulin × 192.)

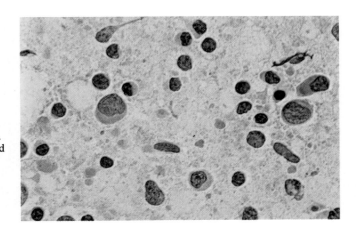

Fig. 6.6. **Reticulosarcoma.** Same case as in *Figs.* 6.3 and 6.4. Smear showing polymorphism of tumour cells. Nuclei tend to be partly indented; nuclear chromatin is stippled. (HE × 480.)

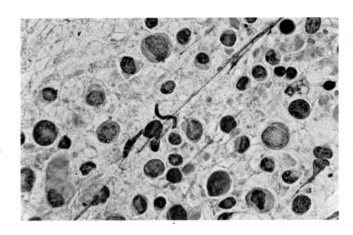

Fig. 6.7. **Reticulosarcoma.**
Same case as in *Figs*. 6.3,
6.4 and 6.6. Smear: cellular
and nuclear polymorphism
is well shown. Typical
mature cell of histiocytic
type shown bottom left,
with small rather condensed
nucleus and abundant
cytoplasm. Such cells
contain diastase-resistant
PAS-positive material and
acid phosphatase.
(HE × 480.)

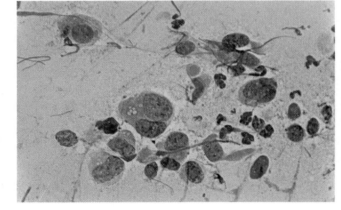

Fig. 6.8. **Reticulosarcoma.**
Another case. Smear
showing polymorphic
cytology. Binucleate tumour
cells and scattered
granulocytes are present.
Some nuclei are reniform;
stippled nuclear chromatin.
(HE × 480.)

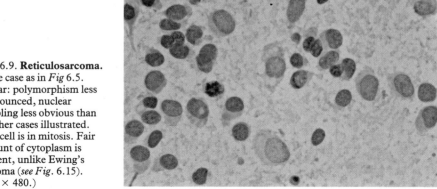

Fig. 6.9. **Reticulosarcoma.**
Same case as in *Fig* 6.5.
Smear: polymorphism less
pronounced, nuclear
stippling less obvious than
in other cases illustrated.
One cell is in mitosis. Fair
amount of cytoplasm is
present, unlike Ewing's
sarcoma (*see Fig*. 6.15).
(HE × 480.)

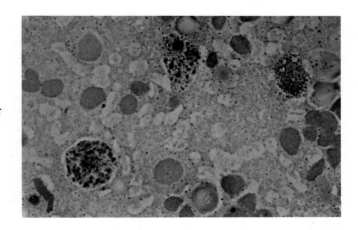

Fig. 6.10.
Reticulosarcoma. Another
case. Smear showing acid
phosphatase in histiocytic
cells with abundant
cytoplasm and condensed
nuclei. These cells also
contain diastase-resistant
PAS-positive material.
(Acid phosphatase
preparation × 480.)

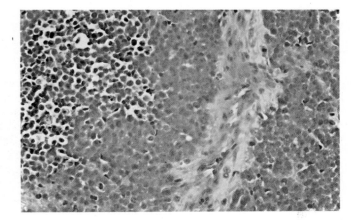

Fig. 6.11. **Ewing's tumour.**
Histology showing closely
packed round tumour cells
on either side of a blood
vessel. Beyond the
perivascular cuff,
degeneration and necrosis
has occurred. (HE × 192.)

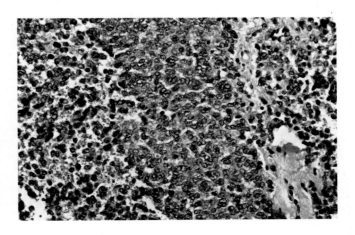

Fig. 6.12. **Ewing's tumour.**
Another case. Paravascular
band of viable tumour, with
degeneration and necrosis
beyond. The clustering of
small groups of cells is
clearly shown; pseudo-
rosettes are seen in this type
of tumour. (HE × 192.)

tumour cells. Diastase-resistant PAS-positive material may be present in a fair proportion of the more mature tumour cells (*Fig.* 6.4).

Cytological smears from reticulosarcoma (*Figs.* 6.6–9) display the usual cytological features observed in the histological sections, but in fuller detail and with greater clarity. There is appreciable variation in cell shape and size, mainly as a reflection of the stage of development and maturation of the individual cells. Occasional cells may have highly hyperchromatic nuclei and scanty cytoplasm, and these are presumably undifferentiated 'blastic' precursors of the more typical lesional cells. Some cells are of intermediate form, having ovoid or reniform nuclei with nucleoli and stippled chromatin. Their cytoplasm is more abundant than in the 'blastic' cells. Yet more mature cells have smaller, partly condensed nuclei, and often abundant cytoplasm; they conform closely to histiocytes, have PAS-positive material in their cytoplasm and are acid phosphatase positive (*Fig.* 6.10). They may show evidence of phagocytic activity, with ingested red cells or nuclear debris in their cytoplasm. Occasional binucleate cells may be present. These should not be mistaken for Reed–Sternberg cells, because they are smaller and lack the prominent large nucleoli typically found in Hodgkin's disease. Mitoses are easy to find but are mostly of normal type. A variable number of mature lymphocytes, and sometimes granulocytes or eosinophils, may accompany some, but not all, reticulosarcomas. Glycogen is not demonstrable in any of the tumour cells.

EWING'S TUMOUR

It is impossible to give a succinct definition or characterization of Ewing's tumour or to be sure of its precise histogenetic derivation. In lieu of a definition, one is usually forced to give a lengthy description of its typical histological features. Speculation as to its possible derivation does not particularly help our understanding of this tumour; it is uncertain whether it is derived from the endothelium, as originally suggested (Ewing, 1921), from the mesenchymal connective tissue framework of the bone-marrow (Dahlin, 1967; Lichtenstein, 1972) or from immature reticulum cells and haemopoietic stem cells and thus related to the malignant lymphomas (Friedman and Gold, 1968; Kadin and Bensch, 1971).

A typical example of Ewing's tumour shows the following histological features.
   a. It is composed of fairly closely packed round or ovoid cells (*Figs.* 6.11 and 6.12) with scanty cytoplasm and ill-defined margins, often giving the impression of a syncytial or symplasmic arrangement. There is little fibrous or fibrillar stroma and the blood vessels within the tumour are fairly widely separated, forming a broad latticed framework. Because of this relative lack of supporting stroma, much of the tumour forms a dense cellular suspension in which small groups of cells may cluster together (*Fig.* 6.12), tending to produce distinct pseudo-rosettes. Because of the wide separation of the blood vessels, the tumour tends to undergo bands or islands of degeneration and necrosis beyond a cuff of variable width around the blood vessels (*Figs.* 6.11– 14). Necrosis may be very extensive, so that strings of blood vessels with a thin rim of tumour may appear to course through wide spaces littered with necrotic cells and cellular debris.
   b. Glycogen is usually demonstrable (Schajowicz, 1959) in viable non-degenerate tumour cells (*Fig.* 6.13); hence it is usually limited to tumour immediately bordering the blood vessels. Away from the blood vessels and approaching the zones of relative ischaemia, the glycogen disappears from the tumour cells.

c. The reticulin structure (*Fig.* 6.14) is extremely sparse, being mainly confined to the vascular network, i.e. it is of a 'vascular' pattern. It is thus seen as a widely separated lattice, with little or no reticulin in between.

The most concise categorization we can give of typical Ewing's tumour is: a malignant round cell tumour of a certain histological appearance, as described above, which is glycogen-positive and reticulin-sparse.

Cytologically (*Fig.* 6.15) the characteristic undegenerate cell of Ewing's tumour presents an essentially monomorphic picture, with round or ovoid nuclei lacking hyperchromatism or pleomorphism, in which the chromatin is fine and fairly diffusely dispersed; nucleoli are very fine or indiscernible. Mitoses can be found and are usually of normal configuration. Binucleate or multinucleate cells are not seen. The cytoplasm is sparse, with ill-defined margins, and tends to disrupt, so that bare nuclei abound. Syncytial cells cannot be identified, despite the contrary impression in histological sections. Degenerate cells tend to be somewhat smaller, with smaller darker condensed nuclei. Necrotic cells are greatly shrunken, with small pyknotic, karyolytic or smudgy nuclei. This admixture of undegenerate, degenerating and necrotic cells should not be taken as a form of polymorphism— the tumour is essentially a monomorphic one.

The demonstration of glycogen in smears (*Fig.* 6.16) is surprisingly and disappointingly inconstant, and may be limited to a relatively small percentage of the cell population. This is true even in material which, in histological sections, contains much glycogen. Alkaline phosphatase is said to be present (Gomori, 1946) in the cells of Ewing's tumour, but in our experience this enzyme is more often than not absent or minimal.

Smears from Ewing's tumour can sometimes be disappointing because degenerate and necrotic cells may predominate, even when apparently viable cellular parts of the tumour have been selected for smearing. It would seem that the viable cells are more cohesive than the degenerate and necrotic cells and hence less easily dislodged in the preparation of smears. This behaviour may also explain the relative scarcity of glycogen-positive cells in many smears.

'Atypical Ewing's tumour'

Some examples of apparent Ewing's tumour lack some of the usual characteristics expected from the typical case.

1. The cellular structure may appear atypical, largely because of the preponderance of degenerate and necrotic tumour, so that little remains of the normal pattern one expects from the typical case. The nuclei undergo condensation and pyknosis, the cytoplasm becomes shrunken and eosinophilic, the apparent symplasmia disappears. It is not unusual to find these changes in many small biopsy samples of Ewing's tumour, hindering its confident diagnosis.
2. Glycogen may not be demonstrable. Whether the glycogen is intrinsically lacking from the tumour cells, or its absence is due to widespread degenerative change is often impossible to determine.
3. A relatively brisk reticulin stroma may be present in some atypical cases.

With some cases of malignant round-cell tumour it may be difficult or impossible to decide whether one is dealing with an 'atypical Ewing's tumour' or a reticulosarcoma. One such case (*Figs.* 6.17–19) was classified in this Registry as 'atypical Ewing's tumour', although reservations were expressed as to whether it might be a reticulosarcoma or an intermediate type of sarcoma. Histologically

Fig. 6.13. **Ewing's tumour.**
Same case as in Fig. 6.11.
Perivascular cuff of tumour
with necrosis beyond.
Glycogen is present in viable
tumour cells immediately
bordering the blood vessel.
Apparently viable cells·
bordering the necrotic
tumour are devoid of
glycogen; these cells are
apparently undergoing
degenerative change.
(PAS × 192.)

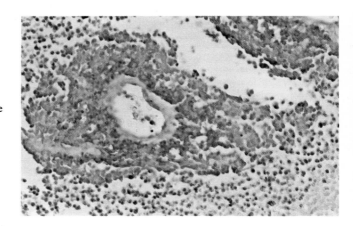

Fig. 6.14. **Ewing's tumour.**
Same case as in Figs. 6.11
and 6.13. Cuff of tumour
surrounding blood vessel,
with necrosis beyond.
Reticulin scanty, mainly
confined to vascular
margins. (Reticulin × 192.)

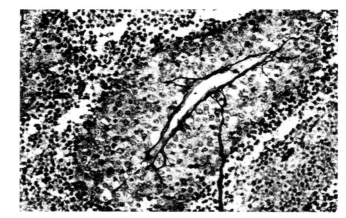

Fig. 6.15. **Ewing's tumour.**
Another case. Smear
showing typical
cytomorphology. Round or
ovoid nuclei. Pale, relatively
diffuse chromatin with only
indistinct stippling, fine
nucleoli. Cytoplasm scanty;
cytoplasmic margins ill-
defined. A cell in mitosis is
present. Degenerate cells
have smaller darker nuclei.
(HE × 480.)

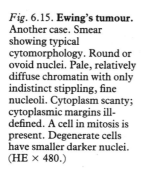

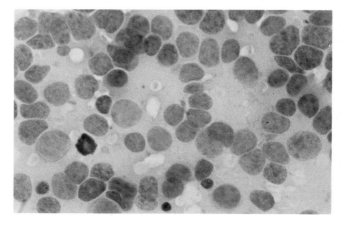

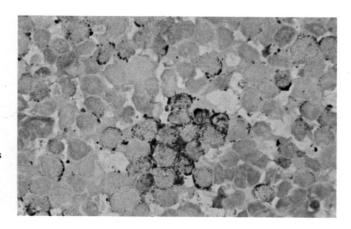

Fig. 6.16. **Ewing's tumour.** Another case. Smear showing glycogen in a proportion of the tumour cells. The relative scantiness of the cytoplasm is shown, as are the cell margins; in HE smears the cytoplasmic borders are very difficult to define. (PAS × 480.)

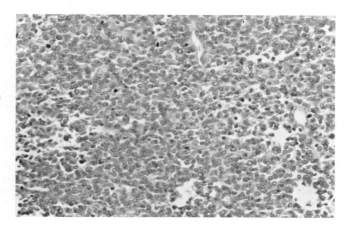

Fig. 6.17. **'Atypical Ewing's tumour'.** Histological pattern resembles Ewing's tumour, but other features of that tumour are lacking. This was classified as 'atypical Ewing's tumour', but might equally be 'atypical reticulosarcoma' or an intermediate form of tumour.

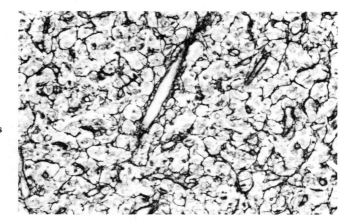

Fig. 6.18. **'Atypical Ewing's tumour'.** Same case as in *Fig.* 6.17. Brisk reticulin stroma, not typical of Ewing's tumour, but in keeping with a reticulosarcoma. (Reticulin × 192.)

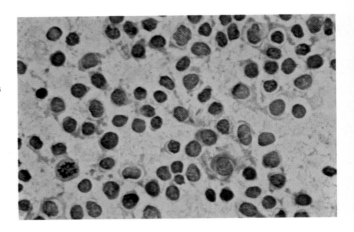

Fig. 6.19. **'Atypical Ewing's tumour'**. Same case as in *Figs.* 6.17 and 6.18. Cytomorphology is not typical of Ewing's tumour, but has some features of reticulosarcoma. Uncertainties, perhaps misdiagnoses, are bound to arise with some cases of 'malignant round-cell tumour'. (HE × 480.)

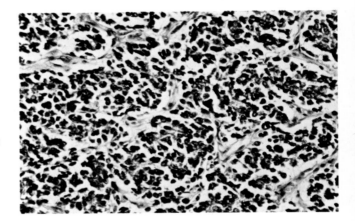

Fig. 6.20. **Metastatic neuroblastoma.** A common histological pattern, with primitive 'blastic' tumour cells having dark hyperchromatic nuclei and scanty cytoplasm. (HE × 192.)

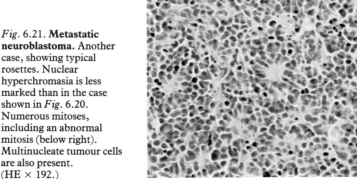

Fig. 6.21. **Metastatic neuroblastoma.** Another case, showing typical rosettes. Nuclear hyperchromasia is less marked than in the case shown in *Fig.* 6.20. Numerous mitoses, including an abnormal mitosis (below right). Multinucleate tumour cells are also present. (HE × 192.)

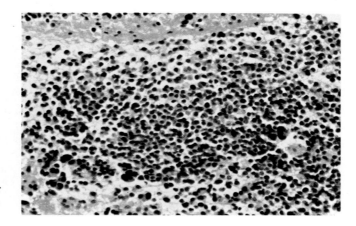

Fig. 6.22. **Metastatic neuroblastoma.** Another case. Another pattern. Nuclear hyperchromasia. Scattered cells with giant or multiple nuclei are present. (HE × 192.)

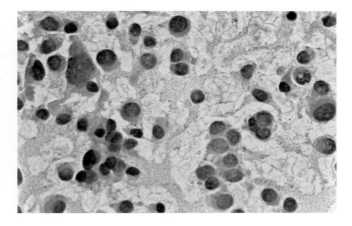

Fig. 6.23. **Metastatic neuroblastoma.** Another case. Smear showing tumour cells with hyperchromatic nuclei and well-defined relatively abundant eosinophilic cytoplasm. A tumour giant-cell with bizarre nucleus is seen top left. Although this case was initially diagnosed histologically as Ewing's tumour, the cytomorphology is totally wrong for Ewing's tumour. (HE × 480.)

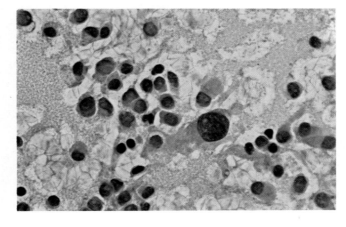

Fig. 6.24. **Metastatic neuroblastoma.** Same case as in *Fig.* 6.23. Smear showing nuclear hyperchromasia and pleomorphism, including a cell with a giant nucleus. None of these features is expected in Ewing's tumour. (HE × 480.)

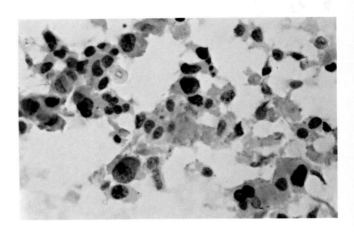

Fig. 6.25. **Metastatic neuroblastoma.** Another case. Smear from needle aspiration biopsy of an osseous metastasis in a patient with retroperitoneal neuroblastoma. Note nuclear pleomorphism and hyperchromasia, numbers of giant nuclei, fairly abundant eosinophilic cytoplasm. (HE × 480.)

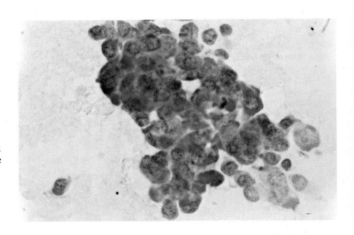

Fig. 6.26. **Metastatic neuroblastoma.** Same case as in *Figs.* 6.23 and 6.24. Smear showing clump of tumour cells rich in glycogen. Up to 20 % of neuroblastomas may contain glycogen, so that this feature does not help in differentiating between Ewing's tumour and neuroblastoma. (PAS × 480.)

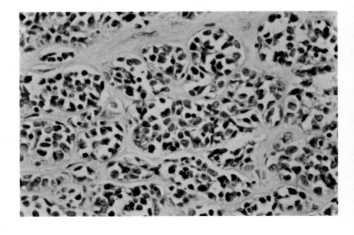

Fig. 6.27. **Metastatic alveolar rhabdomyosarcoma.** Parcelled or 'alveolar' arrangement of round, ovoid and occasional tadpole-shaped cells. (HE × 192.)

Fig. 6.28. **Metastatic alveolar rhabdomyosarcoma.** Same case as in *Fig.* 6.27. Smear showing round or ovoid tumour cells; cytoplasm scanty, nuclear chromatin stippled. In the absence of tadpole-shaped cells, such a field conforms to a 'malignant round-cell tumour'. Ewing's tumour would be ruled out by the nuclear pattern; neuroblastoma by the scanty non-eosinophilic cytoplasm; reticulosarcoma would be favoured. (HE × 480.)

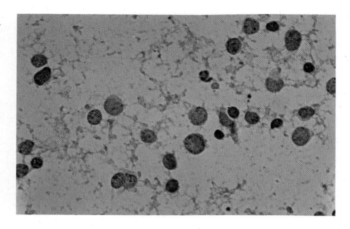

Fig. 6.29. **Metastatic alveolar rhabdomyosarcoma.** Same case as in *Figs.* 6.27 and 6.28. Another field from the smears, showing a tadpole-shaped tumour cell, indicating the diagnosis. (HE × 480.)

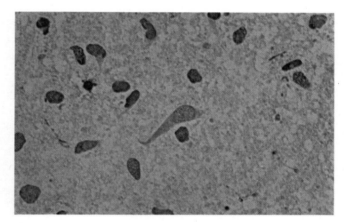

Fig. 6.30. **Plasma-cell myeloma.** Typical histology of well-differentiated tumour. (HE × 307.)

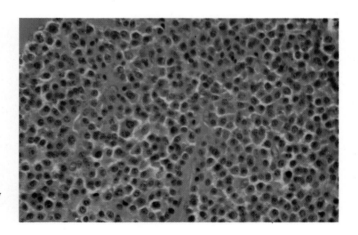

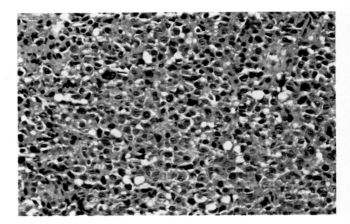

Fig. 6.31. **Plasma-cell myeloma.** A primitive plasma-cell myeloma with considerable pleomorphism. This anaplastic tumour supervened in a patient who had more typical myeloma elsewhere. (HE × 192.)

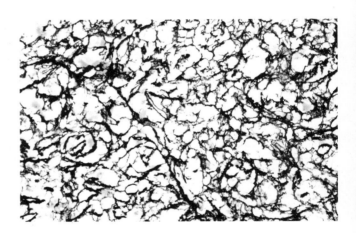

Fig. 6.32. **Plasma-cell myeloma.** Same case as in *Fig.* 6.31. Brisk reticulin pattern. Some conventional plasma-cell myelomas also produce brisk reticulin, although most are reticulin-sparse. (Reticulin × 192.)

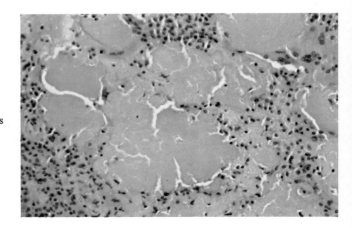

Fig. 6.33. **Plasma-cell myeloma.** A Bence–Jones myeloma producing abundant deposits of 'amyloid' in its stroma. The amyloid in this instance does not give the usual staining characteristics, and the material is presumed to be light-chain protein. Relatively scanty tumour cells may be found in this type of myeloma. (HE × 192.)

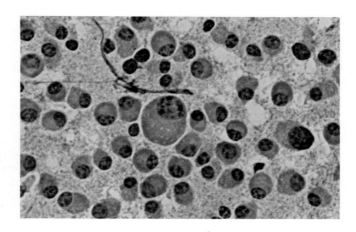

Fig. 6.34. **Plasma-cell myeloma.** Typical cytomorphology with coarsely clumped 'cartwheel' nuclear chromatin. Large cells with giant nuclei present; in other fields mitoses and large cells with multiple nuclei could be found. (HE × 480.)

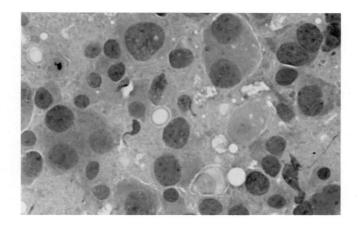

Fig. 6.35. **Plasma-cell myeloma.** Same case as in *Figs.* 6.31 and 6.32. A primitive myeloma with considerable nuclear pleomorphism. Nuclei do not have the clumped chromatin seen in well-differentiated myeloma. (HE × 480.)

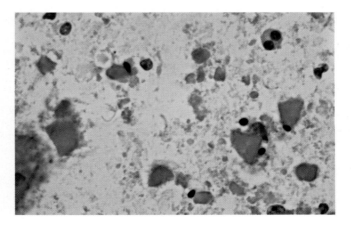

Fig. 6.36. **Plasma-cell myeloma.** Same case as in *Fig.* 6.33. Most of the smeared material represents the amyloid from the tumour stroma, and myeloma cells are extremely scanty. A binucleate myeloma cell is shown here (top right). (HE × 480.)

(*Fig.* 6.17) there is a similarity to Ewing's tumour in HE sections, but the reticulin stroma is fairly brisk (*Fig.* 6.18) and glycogen is absent. Cytologically (*Fig.* 6.19) the cell morphology appears intermediate between typical Ewing's tumour and typical reticulosarcoma. The precise classification of this particular tumour remains debatable. It is salutary to recognize that such cases are bound to arise and that not every malignant round-cell tumour can be neatly placed in a particular category.

METASTATIC NEUROBLASTOMA

Neuroblastoma may present clinically with an osseous metastasis as its first manifestation. Biopsy material from metastatic neuroblastoma is often relatively scanty and may be extensively necrotic, so that the histological diagnosis may have to be a tentative one of a 'malignant round-cell tumour, possibly neuroblastoma', with advice for further investigation, including a search for a possible primary and examination of the urine for catecholamines.

Histologically, the variations which occur with neuroblastoma are shown in (*Figs.* 6.20–22). A common pattern (*Fig.* 6.20) shows heavily hyperchromatic round or oval nuclei with scanty cytoplasm. Typical rosettes (*Fig.* 6.21) may be found, but they are often inconstant and may be absent or difficult to identify in many samples. Some nuclear pleomorphism is detectable in many cases, exceptionally large cells with large polyploid or multiple nuclei being present; mitoses are frequent and abnormal mitoses can be found. In some tumours (*Fig.* 6.22), the cytoplasm may be less scanty and some cells may show abundant cytoplasm with partial differentiation into ganglion cells. In some cases with extensive necrosis viable tumour may only be found in a narrow rim around blood vessels; such a tumour may be difficult to differentiate histologically from Ewing's tumour. Glycogen is present in some neuroblastomas, perhaps up to a quarter of all cases (Arthur et al., 1970; Price, 1973). The reticulin stroma of neuroblastoma is relatively sparse, may be parcelled or predominantly of a 'vascular' pattern. Thus, neither the glycogen content nor the reticulin structure may help in differentiating neuroblastoma from Ewing's tumour.

Cytological smears from neuroblastoma (*Figs.* 6.23–26) show nuclear hyperchromasia, in striking contrast to Ewing's tumour or reticulosarcoma, and there is some variation in nuclear size, with occasional giant or multiple nuclei; the latter are not a feature of Ewing's tumour. The cytoplasmic borders are fairly well defined, in contrast with Ewing's tumour, and the cytoplasm is decidedly eosinophilic, unlike Ewing's tumour or reticulosarcoma. Some smears from neuroblastoma show glycogen in the tumour cells (*Fig.* 6.26). Monoamine oxidase should be demonstrable in most cases of neuroblastoma, but we have not been particularly successful in this in the few cases in which it was tried out.

OTHER METASTATIC EMBRYONAL TUMOURS

It is extremely rare for malignant embryonal tumours other than neuroblastoma to present with osseous metastases. We have come across only one example and this was an alveolar rhabdomyosarcoma (*Fig.* 6.27) with metastases in the tibia, humerus and the skull. Histologically, alveolar rhabdomyosarcoma may show characteristic gland-like spaces lined by rounded, ovoid and some tadpole-shaped cells, and the spaces often contain elongated multinucleate tumour giant-cells. At other times, as in the case illustrated in *Fig.* 6.27, gland-like spaces are absent or ill-distinct and the tumour then shows a parcelled arrangement of round or ovoid

Table 1. Differentiating features of malignant round-cell tumours

	Reticulosarcoma	Ewing's tumour	Neuroblastoma
Cytomorphology	Polymorphic	Monomorphic	Some pleomorphism present
Nuclei	Oval, reniform or grooved. Variable in size and shape. Binucleate cells occur. Chromatin stippled or granular	Round or oval. Uniform size in undegenerate cells. Diffuse fine chromatin. No giant or multiple nuclei	Round or oval. Variable in size. Giant or multiple nuclei occur. Chromatin dark and dense, diffuse or clumped
Cytoplasm	Pale, finely granular. Fair to moderate in amount in juvenile cells; abundant in more mature cells. Cell margins distinct	Pale and uniform. Scanty in amount. Cell margins indistinct	Eosinophilic and uniform. Variable in amount, usually fair to moderate. Cell margins distinct
Glycogen	Absent	Usually present (may be absent in some cases)	Absent in most cases (present in about 20 % of cases)
Acid phosphatase	Present in mature histiocytes	Absent	Absent
Alkaline phosphatase	Absent	Usually absent or minimal	Absent
Diastase-resistant PAS-positive material	Present in mature histiocytes	Absent	Absent
Rosettes	Absent	Pseudo-rosettes may be present	Present (may be absent or difficult to find in many cases)
Reticulin stroma	Abundant (irregular peri-cellular network with some tendency to parcelling)	Sparse (reticulin network usually of 'vascular' pattern)	Sparse (reticulin network may be parcelled or of 'vascular' pattern)

cells with relatively few tadpole-shaped cells and no giant multinucleate cells.

Cytologically, this case showed a predominance of rounded or ovoid tumour cells (*Fig.* 6.28) with scanty cytoplasm and stippled nuclei. The distribution of the nuclear chromatin does not conform to that seen in Ewing's tumour and the absence of eosinophilic cytoplasm renders a diagnosis of metastatic neuroblastoma improbable. The closest approximation is perhaps to reticulosarcoma. However, occasional tadpole-shaped tumour cells (*Fig.* 6.29) are present, ruling out reticulosarcoma and indicating the diagnosis of an embryonal rhabdomyosarcoma.

Differentiation of malignant round-cell tumours

The main differentiating features of the malignant round-cell tumours are given in *Table 1* in summarized form.

PLASMA-CELL MYELOMA

A relatively small proportion of plasma-cell myelomas present primarily via the orthopaedic surgeons, either with an apparently solitary destructive mass in a bone or with a pathological fracture, in which instances biopsy material reaches the bone tumour pathologist.

Histologically (*Fig.* 6.30), plasma-cell myeloma shows a diffuse infiltrate of myeloma cells which retain a distinct, if variable, resemblance to normal plasma cells. Well-differentiated examples show all the characteristics of plasma cells, including the coarsely clumped—so-called 'cartwheel'—nuclear chromatin, eccentric round nucleus, ovoid shape of the cell, pyroninophilia and paranuclear Hof. Nevertheless, even the well-differentiated tumour shows some variation in nuclear size and contains multinucleate cells. Less well-differentiated examples fall into one of two groups. In one, the tumour cells are fairly uniform but of primitive type, with open finely stippled nuclei and prominent nucleoli, lacking the coarse clumping of nuclear chromatin. This type requires differentiation from undifferentiated round-celled metastatic carcinoma, for instance some prostatic carcinomas and seminomas. In the other type, which might be called a 'plasma-cell sarcoma' (*Figs.* 6.31 and 6.32), there is considerable cellular and nuclear pleomorphism, the tumour cells are exceptionally large, with hyperchromatic nuclei; cells with giant or multiple nuclei are frequent and may be of bizarre appearance. This type may require differentiation from pleomorphic reticulosarcoma.

Most examples of plasma-cell myeloma show relatively scanty reticulin, but a small percentage, including well-differentiated tumours, may be reticulin-rich. A few tumours, in our experience light-chain-secreting or Bence–Jones myelomas, produce abundant amorphous lightly eosinophilic material which collects in broad irregular islands and bands throughout the tumour stroma (*Fig.* 6.33). This material looks like, and indeed may be a form of, amyloid but it often does not stain positively with the usual staining techniques for amyloid; it is probably an accumulation of light-chain protein in the tissues.

Smears from plasma-cell myeloma (*Figs.* 6.34–36) reflect the variations of cell morphology which have been mentioned in the histological description given above. Indeed, plasma-cell myeloma is the easiest of all tumours to diagnose in smeared preparations and special cytochemical stains add little further information of any diagnostic importance. Methyl-green-pyronin will demonstrate the pyroninophilia, but we rarely use it. The tumour cells are extremely rich in beta-glucuronidase, but this enzyme is all too often abundantly present in the cells of many other tumours, including metastatic carcinomas. It should be said, however, that a suspected myeloma which is devoid of this enzyme is unlikely to be myeloma.

Cytodiagnostic problems with smears of plasma-cell myeloma may occasionally arise. Necrotic or highly degenerate tumour may lack the usual distinguishing features. Tumours which have been extensively replaced by amyloid may yield only scanty recognizable tumour cells, so that a confident cytological diagnosis may be impossible (*Fig.* 6.36). Certain carcinomas may resemble primitive myeloma, for instance anaplastic prostatic carcinoma and seminoma. Seminoma may present the added problem that it may show an abundance of superimposed non-neoplastic

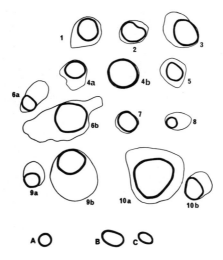

Line drawings of representative cells from malignant round-cell tumours and plasma-cell myeloma. Osteoclast and small lymphocyte nuclei are also given for comparison; a normal plasma cell is also shown.

These and all other line drawings in this volume have been drawn at the same magnification.

1. Lymphoblastic lymphosarcoma (large cell or lymphoblast from *Fig.* 6.2). The nuclear size in the small lymphocytes in this smear is similar to that of normal small lymphocytes.
2. Reticulosarcoma (cell from *Fig.* 6.6).
3. Reticulosarcoma (cell from *Fig.* 6.9).
4. Ewing's tumour (cells from *Fig.* 6.15):
    4a: Degenerate cell. Nucleus in degenerate Ewing cell shrinks, hence the cytoplasm appears more abundant than is usual with undegenerate cell.
    4b: Undegenerate cell. Nucleus of undegenerate Ewing cell is larger than the nuclei of lymphoblastic lymphosarcoma or reticulosarcoma; it is also larger than the average nucleus in neuroblastoma. Cytoplasm is barely discernible.
5. 'Atypical Ewing's tumour' (cell from *Fig.* 6.19). Small nuclear size and fair amount of cytoplasm indicate that the diagnosis of Ewing's tumour in this case is probably spurious.
6. Neuroblastoma (cells from *Fig.* 6.24):
    6a: Average cell. Nucleus small, only slightly larger than nucleus of lymphocyte; relatively abundant cytoplasm.
    6b: Large cell. Nucleus large, rather larger than nucleus of undegenerate Ewing cell; cytoplasm abundant.
7. Alveolar rhabdomyosarcoma ('round cell' from *Fig.* 6.28). Relatively small nucleus, relatively scanty cytoplasm.
8. Non-neoplastic plasma-cell from chronic osteomyelitis (cell from *Fig.* 8.13, Chapter 8).
9. Plasma-cell myeloma, average case (cells from *Fig.* 6.34):
    9a: Average cell.
    9b: Large cell.
10. Plasma-cell myeloma, poorly-differentiated case (cells from *Fig.* 6.35):
    10a: Large cell.
    10b: Average cell.
A. Nucleus of small lymphocyte.
B. Nucleus of juvenile osteoclast.
C. Nucleus of mature osteoclast.

Nuclear size in non-Hodgkin malignant lymphoma and Ewing's tumour is best compared with that of a normal small lymphocyte; they are all much larger, the largest being those in Ewing's tumour.

Nuclear size in plasma-cell myeloma is best compared with that of a normal plasma cell. The average myeloma-cell nucleus is larger than that of a normal plasma cell, but the nuclei of some tumour cells are very much larger.

plasma cells. Caution is also required with the so-called 'pseudo-myeloma', which is a chronic infective lesion very heavily infiltrated with plasma cells. In pseudo-myeloma the plasma cells are fully mature and many will contain Russell bodies; there is also a sprinkling of lymphocytes and granulocytes. Mitoses are absent. These features should help in its differentiation from plasma-cell myeloma.

The nuclear size in representative cells from various 'malignant round-cell tumours' and plasma-cell myeloma is outlined above in black-and-white tracings (p. 119), drawn at the same magnification.

References

Arthur T.F., Bennett M.H., Jelliffe A.M. et al. (1970) Small round-cell tumours of bone. In: Jelliffe A.M. and Strickland B. (ed.), *Symposium Ossium*. Edinburgh and London, Livingstone, p. 186.

Dahlin D.C. (1967) *Bone Tumors*, 2nd ed. Springfield, Ill., Thomas, p. 186.

Ewing J. (1921) Diffuse endothelioma of bone. *Proc. N.Y. Pathol. Soc. 21*, 17.

Friedman B. and Gold H. (1968) Ultrastructure of Ewing's sarcoma of bone. *Cancer 22*, 307.

Gall E.A. and Mallory T.B. (1942) Malignant lymphoma: a clinico-pathologic survey of 618 cases. *Am. J. Pathol. 18*, 381.

Gomori G. (1946) The study of enzymes in tissue sections. *Am. J. Clin. Pathol. 16*, 347.

Kadin M.E. and Bensch K.G. (1971) On the origin of Ewing's tumor. *Cancer 27*, 257.

Lichtenstein L. (1972) *Bone Tumors*, 4th ed. St Louis, Mosby, p. 258.

Parker F. jun. and Jackson H. jun. (1939) Primary reticulum cell sarcoma of bone. *Surg. Gynecol. Obstet. 68*, 45.

Price C.H.G. (1973) A critique of Ewing's tumour of bone. In: Price C.H.G. and Ross F.G.M. (ed.), *Bone—Certain Aspects of Neoplasia*. London, Butterworths, p. 181.

Schajowicz, F. (1959) Ewing's sarcoma and reticulum-cell sarcoma of bone, with special reference to the histochemical demonstration of glycogen as an aid to differential diagnosis. *J. Bone Joint Surg. 41-A*, 349.

Chapter 7

Metastatic Carcinoma

In dealing with biopsy material from suspected metastatic carcinoma the pathologist has to confirm the presence of a malignant lesion, to decide that it is of epithelial origin and not a primary sarcoma of bone, and to try and determine, if possible, the probable source of the metastasis. With adequate sampling cytological smears will readily confirm the presence of malignancy, permit the differentiation of carcinoma from sarcoma in most cases (the exceptions being some anaplastic carcinomas which could be confused with malignant round-cell tumours), and in some cases establish the probable origin of the metastasis.

Whereas we consider cytological smears superior to cryostat sections for the rapid diagnosis of bone sarcomas, we feel the converse is usually true with metastatic carcinoma. This is because the characteristic structural organization of epithelial tumours, which is readily identifiable in sections, cannot be visualized in smears. Nevertheless, if cytology is to be applied to the study of bone tumours, the cytodiagnostician must be fully conversant with the cytology of all tumours which may be present in bone, including metastatic carcinoma.

The following criteria assist in the identification of metastatic carcinoma:

1. First and foremost, the definite tendency to circumscribed clumping of the tumour cells, best seen with low-power scanning of the smears. In addition, regular rows of cells can usually be found in smears of adenocarcinomas.

2. Cytoplasmic differentiation, when present, is of great value in the recognition of metastatic carcinoma; for instance, squamous differentiation with epidermoid carcinomas, secretory activity with mucus-secreting adenocarcinomas, clear-cell change with glycogen accumulation in renal cortical carcinomas. Demonstration of melanin pigment would establish a metastatic tumour as malignant melanoma. The cytoplasmic configuration itself, for instance tall columnar cells with basal nuclei or the presence of brush or striated borders, can be of diagnostic value.

3. In general, cytochemistry is of little assistance in the identification of carcinoma cells. For instance, a confident diagnosis of prostatic carcinoma can be made if malignant epithelial cells are rich in acid phosphatase, and their enzyme activity is undiminished by incubation with 0·5 % formaldehyde but is inhibited by incubation with M/100 tartrate. Alkaline phosphatase may be demonstrable in a small proportion of carcinomas, including some bladder, gastric and mammary tumours. Beta-glucuronidase is found in most carcinomas, but its demonstration is not of any special diagnostic significance. PAS, with and without diastase, is useful in the demonstration of mucin and glycogen: diastase-resistant PAS +ve globules are characteristically present in mucus-producing adenocarcinomas and diastase-labile PAS +ve glycogen is abundantly found in clear-cell carcinomas of the renal cortex.

4. Nuclear characteristics are not particularly reliable in deciding whether a malignant smear is carcinomatous or sarcomatous, since individual tumours can vary considerably in this respect. As a general rule, nuclei of carcinomas tend to have finer chromatin than sarcomas, greater uniformity of nuclear size, and less tendency to giant or multinucleate tumour cells. The exceptions to this broad rule are, however, numerous and we have learnt to place little reliance on nuclear appearances in this context.

Representative examples will be presented below to illustrate the main cytological groups encountered in smears of metastatic carcinoma.

CARCINOMAS WITH SQUAMOUS DIFFERENTIATION

Smears from metastatic epidermoid carcinomas (*Figs.* 7.1–3), unless completely anaplastic and undifferentiated, show numbers of squamous cells with varying degrees of keratinization. The nuclei of the mature keratinized squamous cells are smaller and pyknotic, in comparison with the less differentiated or less mature tumour cells; their cytoplasm tends to be abundant and increasingly eosinophilic with the degree of keratinization. Granular stipples of glycogen may be present in the cytoplasm. Occasionally, prickle-cells can be identified, with intercellular bridges between adjoining cells.

Demonstration of squamous differentiation in a smear usually, but not necessarily always, indicates an origin from epidermoid epithelium, including metaplastic bronchial epithelium. Occasionally, such cells may be found in smears of carcinomas of urothelial or glandular origin, for instance vesical, endometrial and mammary carcinomas, in which the malignant epithelium itself has undergone squamous metaplasia.

MUCUS-SECRETING ADENOCARCINOMAS

Intra-cytoplasmic globules of mucin are readily demonstrable in smears of mucus-producing adenocarcinomas (*Figs.* 7.4–6). The globule is often single; it may be relatively small or may be larger than the nucleus, displacing the latter to produce a 'signet-ring cell'. The mucin globule can be seen quite easily in HE smears, but is most clearly demonstrated in PAS smears after digestion with diastase.

Cytological identification of mucus-producing carcinoma cells does not permit one to establish the primary source, but helps to narrow down the field to known sites of such carcinomas.

COLUMNAR-CELL ADENOCARCINOMA

Certain well-differentiated tubular, tubulo-papillary or papillary cystic adenocarcinomas, including some types arising from the ovaries, gallbladder, biliary or pancreatic ducts, small intestine and endocervix, produce a regular pattern of tall columnar or 'picket' cells with basal or parabasal nuclei (*Fig.* 7.7).

Cytological smears from such carcinomas (*Fig.* 7.8) show the characteristic columnar shape of the tumour cell and the relatively basal location of the nucleus. The nuclei are often small and of uniform ovoid shape. With an extra-osseous lesion the malignancy of such cells might be open to question in view of their relatively bland cytomorphology, but in an intra-osseous tumour there can be no doubt of their malignant nature.

MUCO-EPIDERMOID CARCINOMA

On occasions, both squamous and mucus-secretory differentiation can be found in smears of a metastatic carcinoma, permitting a cytological diagnosis of muco-epidermoid carcinoma (*Figs.* 7.9–12). In the example illustrated, the muco-epidermoid nature of the tumour was more immediately obvious in the smears than in the histological sections stained with HE. Muco-epidermoid carcinomas may originate at various sites, including the salivary glands, breast and bronchi.

CLEAR-CELL CARCINOMA OF KIDNEY
Smears showing tumour cells with abundant pale or lightly granular cytoplasm, containing glycogen, have in our experience usually proved to be renal cortical adenocarcinomas or 'hypernephromas' (*Figs.* 7.13–15). Lipid is also demonstrable in some of the tumour cells. We have not yet come across non-renal metastatic clear-cell carcinoma, e.g. of the lung, and therefore have no experience of its specific cytology.

Clear-cell carcinoma of the kidney is sometimes said to require differentiation from chordoma the cells of which also contain glycogen. Chordoma, however, contains mucin in many of its cells, often in huge amounts as in the bloated physaliphorous cells (*Figs.* 3.41 and 3.42). Mucin is not found in the clear cells of renal cortical adenocarcinoma and we do not consider that the two conditions should be confused with one another.

TRANSITIONAL-CELL (UROTHELIAL) CARCINOMA
Osseous metastases from vesical and other urothelial carcinomas usually present a pattern that can be recognized both histologically and cytologically (*Figs.* 7.16–18), and the recognition is often helped by the presence of some squamous metaplasia. The transitional cells are greatly elongated or fusiform, with ovoid nuclei, tend to lie in loose sheets with their long axes orientated in the same direction. A proportion of the cells are rounded, without cytoplasmic prolongations, and some may be squamoid.

PROSTATIC ADENOCARCINOMA
Smears from prostatic carcinoma do not show any cytomorphological characteristics to enable its differentiation from other 'round-cell' carcinomas without cytoplasmic differentiation.

A moderately-differentiated prostatic adenocarcinoma is illustrated in *Figs.* 7.19–21. The tumour cells are uniformly spheroidal with round or slightly ovoid nuclei (*Fig.* 7.20), impossible to tell apart from other well-differentiated adenocarcinomas with rounded or cuboidal cells, for instance follicular carcinoma of the thyroid (*Fig.* 7.26). However, the tumour cells contain formol-resistant tartrate-inhibited acid phosphatase (*Fig.* 7.21), an enzyme characteristic which will help establish the diagnosis of prostatic carcinoma.

A poorly-differentiated prostatic adenocarcinoma is shown in *Figs.* 7.22 and 7.23. Cytomorphologically, this is the type of prostatic carcinoma which may sometimes be mistaken for certain types of plasma-cell myeloma because of the rather eccentric position of the nucleus and the coarse granularity of the nuclear chromatin. 'Indian-file' strings of tumour cells, however, can usually be found in the smears to indicate its epithelial origin, and cytoplasmic acid phosphatase can, of course, be demonstrated.

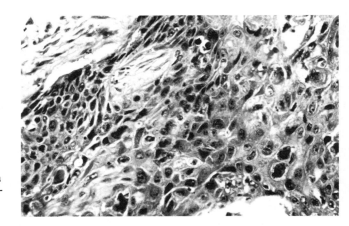

Fig. 7.1. **Squamous carcinoma.** Histologically a well-differentiated and well-preserved tumour. (HE × 192.)

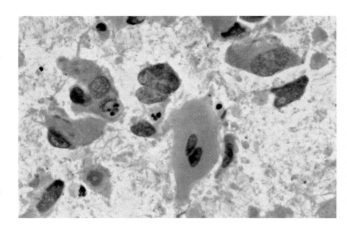

Fig. 7.2. **Squamous carcinoma.** Smear shows keratinized and partly keratinized tumour cells. Cell with fully keratinized orange-red cytoplasm shows nuclear shrinkage and pyknosis. (HE × 480.)

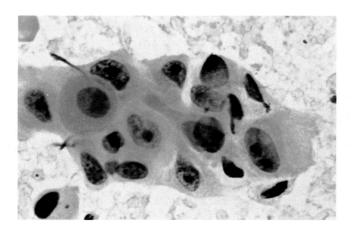

Fig. 7.3. **Squamous carcinoma.** Smear showing cluster of coherent squamous carcinoma cells, some with partial keratinization. (HE × 480.)

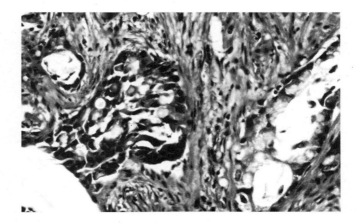

Fig. 7.4. **Mucus-secreting adenocarcinoma.** Glandular spaces lined by cuboidal cells many of which contain secretory vacuoles. Of gastric origin. (HE × 192.)

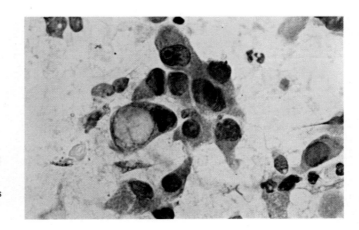

Fig. 7.5. **Mucus-secreting adenocarcinoma.** Smear showing group of tumour cells, one of which contains a large secretory vacuole. (HE × 480.)

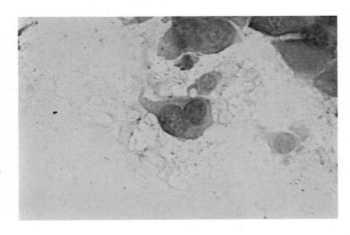

Fig. 7.6. **Mucus-secreting adenocarcinoma.** Smear showing carcinoma cell with vacuole of mucin, rather smaller in size than the nucleus. (PAS-diastase × 480.)

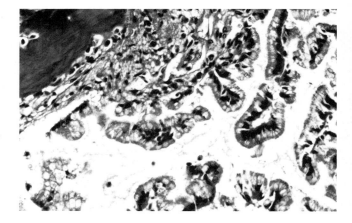

Fig. 7.7. **Columnar-cell adenocarcinoma.**
Histology: papillary tumour with columnar cells having basal nuclei. Origin not positively identified, but necropsy suggested a pancreatic-duct origin. (HE × 192.)

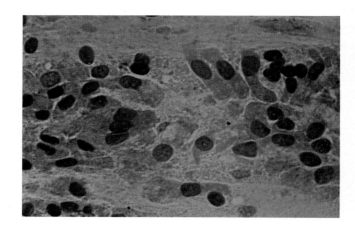

Fig. 7.8. **Columnar-cell adenocarcinoma.** Same case as in *Fig.* 7.7. Smear shows tall columnar cells with basal or parabasal nuclei, faithfully reflecting the structure of the constituent cells as seen in the histological sections. (HE × 480.)

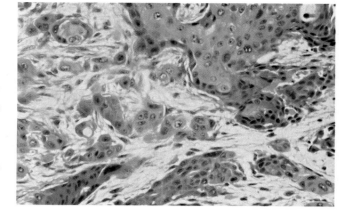

Fig. 7.9. **Muco-epidermoid carcinoma.** Histologically the predominant structure is that of a squamous carcinoma, but on close inspection numbers of vacuolated cells can be seen. The mucus vacuoles in these cells are seen more clearly with PAS (*see Fig.* 7.10). (HE × 192.)

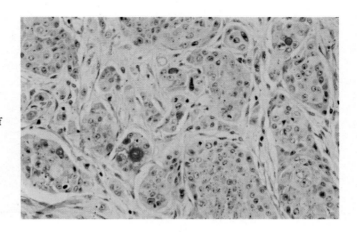

Fig. 7.10. **Muco-epidermoid carcinoma.** Same case as in *Fig.* 7.9. Histology: numerous cells contain rounded vacuoles of mucin. In addition, many cells have PAS positive stipples due to glycogen. These stipples, but not the mucin globules, lost their staining with PAS after digestion with diastase. (PAS × 192.)

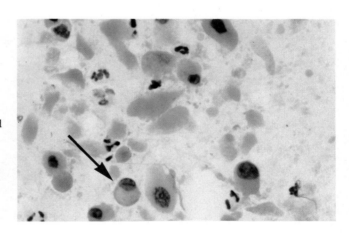

Fig. 7.11. **Muco-epidermoid carcinoma.** Same case as in *Figs.* 7.9 and 7.10. Smear showing numerous squamous cells with condensed pyknotic nuclei; some of the squames are without nuclei. A rounded cell with large secretory vacuole is present (arrowed). (HE × 480.)

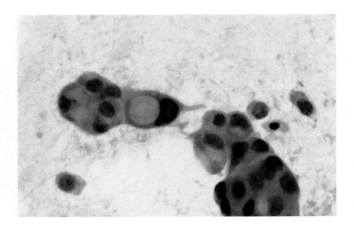

Fig. 7.12. **Muco-epidermoid carcinoma.** Same case as in *Figs.* 7.9–11. Smear shows clusters of cells with glandular characteristics, including a 'signet-ring' cell with large vacuole displacing and indenting the nucleus. (HE × 480.)

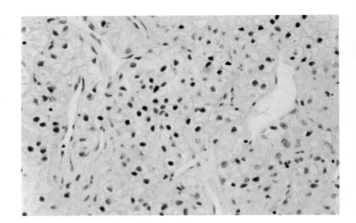

Fig. 7.13. **Clear-cell carcinoma of kidney.** Histology: sheets of rounded and polyhedral cells with clear cytoplasm. (HE × 192.)

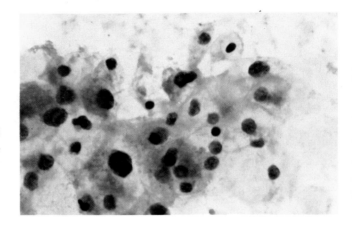

Fig. 7.14. **Clear-cell carcinoma of kidney.** Smear showing cluster of rounded and polyhedral cells. Many cells in this field have granular eosinophilic non-clear cytoplasm. Several cells (at right end of field) have pale cytoplasm, smaller pyknotic nuclei and ill-defined margins. (HE × 480.)

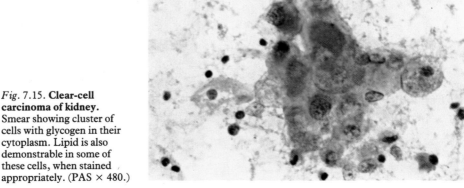

Fig. 7.15. **Clear-cell carcinoma of kidney.** Smear showing cluster of cells with glycogen in their cytoplasm. Lipid is also demonstrable in some of these cells, when stained appropriately. (PAS × 480.)

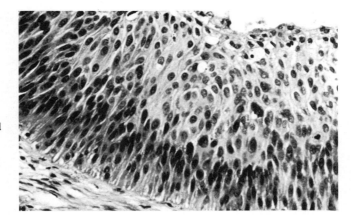

Fig. 7.16. **Transitional-cell (urothelial) carcinoma.** Typical histology with pseudo-stratification of elongated cells. The elongation of the basal cytoplasm is particularly well shown. (HE × 192.)

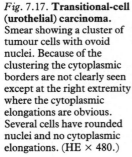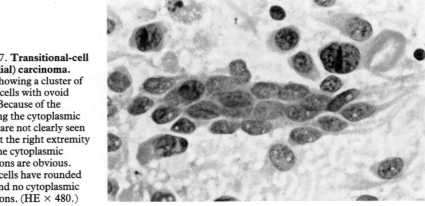

Fig. 7.17. **Transitional-cell (urothelial) carcinoma.** Smear showing a cluster of tumour cells with ovoid nuclei. Because of the clustering the cytoplasmic borders are not clearly seen except at the right extremity where the cytoplasmic elongations are obvious. Several cells have rounded nuclei and no cytoplasmic elongations. (HE × 480.)

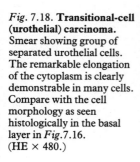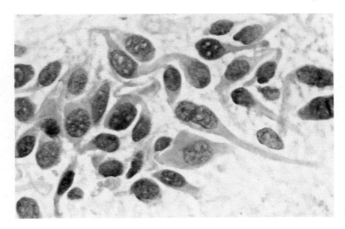

Fig. 7.18. **Transitional-cell (urothelial) carcinoma.** Smear showing group of separated urothelial cells. The remarkable elongation of the cytoplasm is clearly demonstrable in many cells. Compare with the cell morphology as seen histologically in the basal layer in *Fig.*7.16. (HE × 480.)

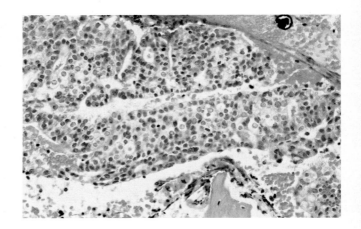

Fig. 7.19. **Prostatic adenocarcinoma.** Moderately-differentiated. Histology shows typical cribriform pattern with cuboidal and spheroidal cells. (HE × 192.)

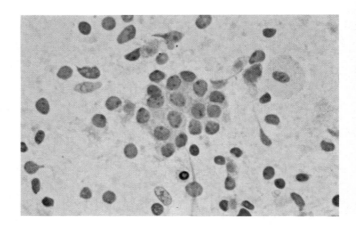

Fig. 7.20. **Prostatic adenocarcinoma.** Same case as in *Fig.* 7.19. Smear shows cluster of spheroidal cells without any distinguishing morphological features. This smear could not be diagnosed as of prostatic origin on cytomorphology alone. (HE × 480.)

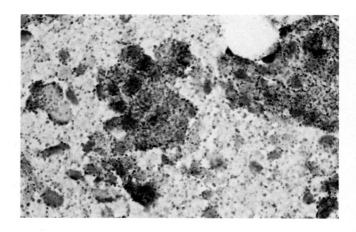

Fig. 7.21. **Prostatic adenocarcinoma.** Same case as in *Figs.* 7.19 and 7.20. Smear shows tumour cells containing acid phosphatase. (Acid phosphatase preparation × 480.)

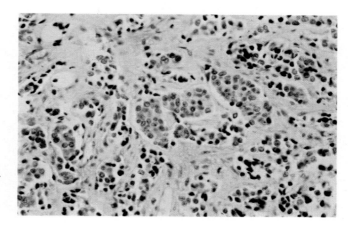

Fig. 7.22. **Prostatic adenocarcinoma.** Histology of rather poorly-differentiated tumour. (HE × 192.)

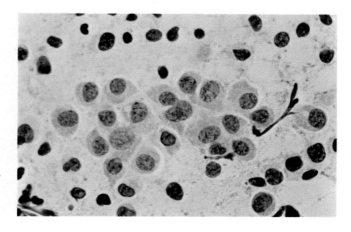

Fig. 7.23. **Prostatic adenocarcinoma.** Same case as in *Fig.* 7.22. Smear shows cells larger than in case seen in *Figs.* 7.19–21, with granular stippled nuclear chromatin. May resemble types of myeloma lacking typical coarse granularity of the nucleus or the characteristic cytoplasmic paranuclear Hof. (HE × 480.)

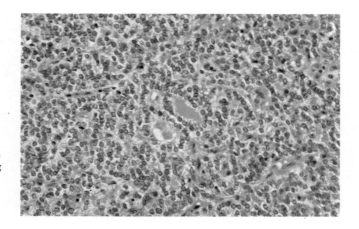

Fig. 7.24. **Follicular carcinoma of thyroid.** Histology of moderately differentiated tumour. Two obvious follicles, containing eosinophilic colloid material, are demonstrable at centre of field. (HE × 192.)

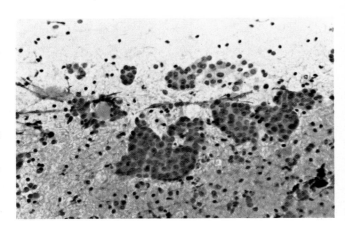

Fig. 7.25. **Follicular carcinoma of thyroid.** Low-power view of smear, showing the discrete circumscribed clumping of tumour cells which is characteristic of carcinomas. Near top left, cells are clustered around amorphous eosinophilic material which could be thyroid secretion from one of the follicles; this latter observation is purely an inference drawn from subsequent knowledge of the histology. (HE × 192.)

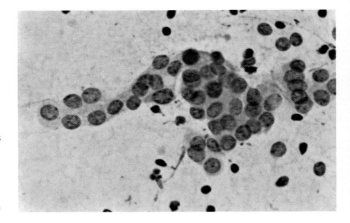

Fig. 7.26. **Follicular carcinoma of thyroid.** Smear showing a cluster of spheroidal or low cuboidal cells. The clear-cut linear arrangement of the cells is obviously seen on both sides and below the main clump. Cytology permits only its identification as a spheroidal-cell carcinoma and gives no indication of a thyroid origin. (HE × 480.)

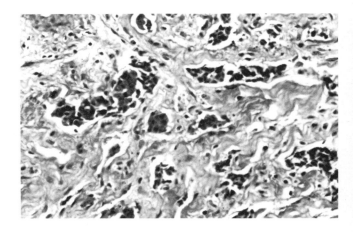

Fig. 7.27. **Mammary carcinoma.** Histology of metastasis from a spheroidal-cell carcinoma with scirrhous stroma. (HE × 192.)

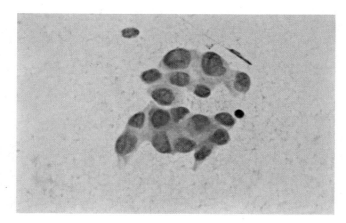

Fig. 7.28. **Mammary carcinoma.** Smear shows cluster of tumour cells, with tendency to linear arrangement. Cytology does not permit precise identification as a mammary carcinoma. (HE × 480.)

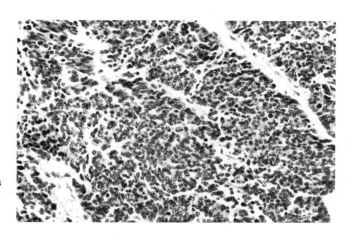

Fig. 7.29. **Oat-cell carcinoma of lung.** Histology: broad strands and clusters of ovoid cells with abundant mitoses. This pattern may be mistaken for Ewing's tumour. (HE × 192.)

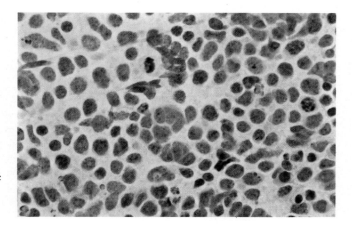

Fig. 7.30. **Oat-cell carcinoma of lung.** Smear shows tumour cells with oval or rounded nuclei and scanty cytoplasm; several mitoses are present. The cells are smaller than those of Ewing's tumour, the nuclei more hyperchromatic and no glycogen is demonstrable in the cytoplasm. (HE × 480.)

CARCINOMAS WITHOUT SPECIFIC CYTOMORPHOLOGICAL OR CYTOCHEMICAL FEATURES

Certain metastatic carcinomas, including both poorly-differentiated and well differentiated forms, lack specific cytomorphological or cytochemical characteristics, as in the groups described above, to permit their cytological identification. A necessarily limited selection of these will be given below.

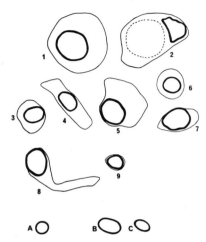

Line drawings of representative cells from metastatic carcinomas. Osteoclast and small lymphocyte nuclei are also given for comparison.

These and all other line drawings in this volume have been drawn at the same magnification.

This particular illustration has been included merely to provide a comparison for the line drawings in the previous chapters. Nuclear size is not, in itself, of particular importance in the assessment of metastatic carcinomas in bone.

1. Squamous carcinoma (cell from *Fig.* 7.3).
2. Mucus-producing adenocarcinoma (cell from *Fig.* 7.5).
3. Prostatic adenocarcinoma (cell from *Fig.* 7.23).
4. Columnar-cell adenocarcinoma (cell from *Fig.* 7.8).
5. Clear-cell carcinoma of kidney (cell from *Fig.* 7.14).
6. Follicular carcinoma of thyroid (cell from *Fig.* 7.26).
7. Carcinoma of breast (cell from *Fig.* 7.28).
8. Transitional-cell carcinoma of bladder (cell from *Fig.* 7.18).
9. Oat-cell carcinoma of lung (cell from *Fig.* 7.30).
A. Nucleus of small lymphocyte.
B. Nucleus of juvenile osteoclast.
C. Nucleus of mature osteoclast.

Follicular carcinoma of thyroid

This is clearly identifiable in histological sections (*Fig.* 7.24). Cytological smears will demonstrate a metastatic carcinoma with spheroidal or cuboidal cells (*Figs.* 7.25 and 7.26). The clumping or circumscribed clustering of tumour cells, characteristic of carcinoma, is clearly shown in a low-power view (*Fig.* 7.25). At high magnification (*Fig.* 7.26) the definite tendency to linear arrangement of the carcinoma cells can be seen. On cytomorphological criteria it would be impossible to decide the site of origin of the tumour. Patchy eosinophilic secretion, presumably derived from the thyroid follicles, can be seen in the background of some such smears.

Carcinoma of breast

Cytological smears from the usual scirrhous spheroidal-cell carcinoma of the breast (*Figs.* 7.27 and 7.28) yield clusters and strings of rounded cells which permit no more than the diagnosis of an unspecified spheroidal-cell carcinoma.

Oat-cell carcinoma of lung

Cytological smears from oat-cell carcinoma of the lung (*Figs.* 7.29 and 7.30) show rounded and ovoid cells with hyperchromatic nuclei and scanty cytoplasm which may prove difficult to differentiate from some primary 'malignant round-cell tumours' of bone, especially 'atypical Ewing's tumour'. In our experience, the most reliable guide in differentiating oat-cell carcinoma from 'malignant round-cell tumour' of bone is the presence of 'Indian-file' strings or sharply circumscribed clumps of tumour cells.

Outline black-and-white tracings are given opposite, comparing the nuclear size in various examples of metastatic carcinoma.

Chapter 8

Histiocytosis X and Inflammatory Lesions

Pathological confirmation of these conditions is usually required even when their nature may be suspected on clinical and radiological grounds. In practice, they may sometimes be difficult to differentiate, before pathological examination, from a variety of benign and malignant bone lesions. Indeed, many of the examples selected to illustrate this chapter were not confidently diagnosed before biopsy.

HISTIOCYTOSIS X

This group includes eosinophilic granuloma, Letterer–Siwe disease and Hand–Christian–Schüller disease. In all these conditions the primary and essential process is that of histiocytic proliferation, believed to be due to some unusual infective agent the nature of which has not, so far, been determined. The clinical and histological variations in Histiocytosis X depend on (1) whether the lesions are confined to bone or disseminated throughout the body, and on (2) the duration or chronicity of the lesions.

Eosinophilic granuloma is confined to one or more bones, and may be acute or chronic. Letterer–Siwe disease and Hand–Christian–Schüller disease are the acute and chronic forms of disseminated Histiocytosis X.

The duration of the disease process has a bearing on both the clinical and histological features of Histiocytosis X. The younger or more recent lesions display active juvenile histiocytes; in the older or senescent lesions, the constituent histiocytes tend to undergo increasing lipid accumulation and become 'foam cells'. Eosinophilic granuloma often presents with active juvenile histiocytic proliferation, but sometimes aged lesions with extensive foam-cell change may be encountered. Since eosinophilic granuloma is localized to bone, the actual age of the lesion does not materially affect the clinical progress with its good prognosis. In disseminated Histiocytosis X, the clinical picture as well as the histological appearances are influenced by the tempo of the disease process. In Letterer–Siwe disease the progress is rapid and usually fatal and the histological picture is dominated by active proliferation of juvenile histiocytes. In Hand–Christian–Schüller disease the clinical course is long-drawn out and the lesional histiocytes are predominantly mature or senescent, so that the histological picture appears 'xanthomatous'.

There are occasions in which a patient with an apparently solitary eosinophilic granuloma subsequently develops further intra-osseous lesions. Intra-osseous Histiocytosis X may subsequently manifest extra-osseous disease. An occasional case of disseminated Histiocytosis X in infancy, suspected to be Letterer–Siwe disease, may enter a chronic phase with long survival. Examples of these variations of progression have been recorded in this Registry.

Letterer–Siwe disease is usually dealt with primarily by the general or paediatric histopathologist, since its biopsy is mainly obtained from extra-osseous lesions. We have no example on record in this Registry. Several examples of Hand–Christian–Schüller disease have been recorded here but only one example has come to be smeared. Eosinophilic granuloma is the commonest form of Histiocytosis X encountered in orthopaedic practice and most of our smears are accordingly from such cases.

Eosinophilic granuloma

Histologically (*Fig.* 8.1), eosinophilic granuloma shows an admixture of histiocytes and eosinophils, the latter often predominating in focal aggregates. In most cases, the histiocytic component is formed by active juvenile histiocytes, some of which may be multinucleate. Foam-cell change may be found in some cases. Focal necroses may be seen and particularly in such areas Charcot–Leyden crystals may be identifiable (*Fig.* 8.2); these crystals are best demonstrated with PTAH and may be difficult to visualize in routine HE sections. In a proportion of cases a sprinkling of polymorphonuclear leucocytes may also be found and lymphocytic infiltration may occur at and beyond the margins of the lesion. It is important to bear in mind that occasionally chronic osteomyelitic lesions may show abundant eosinophils, but in such instances the lesional infiltrate is much more polymorphic and contains abundant plasma cells, lymphocytes and polymorphonuclear leucocytes.

Cytological smears from eosinophilic granuloma (*Figs.* 8.3 and 8.4) show an admixture of histiocytes and eosinophils. The histiocytes are of normal reactive cytomorphology and do not show the nuclear abnormalities expected in malignant histiocytes. They are mostly mononuclear, but binucleate and multinucleate cells may be found. The eosinophils are readily recognizable by their characteristic refractile acidophil granules; typically they have bilobed nuclei, but unlobed and multilobed forms also occur. In degenerate eosinophils the acidophilic granules may be indistinct, but the cell can still be recognized by its bilobed nucleus.

'Lipogranuloma' and 'xanthoma'

Solitary lesions are sometimes encountered which are exclusively foam-celled and these are usually labelled 'xanthomas', 'lipogranulomas' or 'xanthogranulomas'. Such lesions could well be obsolete eosinophilic granulomas but fibrous lesions also may rarely terminate in such a fashion. Hence the antecendent nature of such lesions cannot always be clearly identified.

Letterer–Siwe disease

Although we have not actually examined cytological smears from Letterer–Siwe disease, we believe—from a comparison of the histology of that disease with that of eosinophilic granuloma—that the cytomorphology of the histiocytes in Letterer–Siwe disease would essentially conform to that seen in eosinophil granuloma.

Hand–Christian–Schüller disease

Occasional examples of Histiocytosis X may show a predominance of foamy histiocytes, with relatively scanty juvenile histiocytes or eosinophils, and this is the usual histological pattern in Hand–Christian–Schüller disease. On the histology and cytology alone, the individual lesion cannot be firmly established as obsolete eosinophilic granuloma or Hand–Christian–Schüller disease. The precise diagnosis will depend on whether or not systematized disease is present.

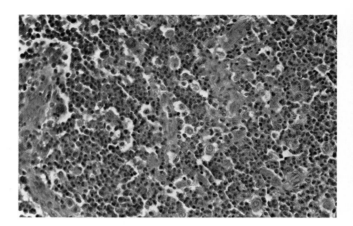

Fig. 8.1. **Histiocytosis X.**
Eosinophilic granuloma.
Typical histology, showing
an admixture of histiocytes
and eosinophils; in places
the eosinophils
predominate. (HE × 192.)

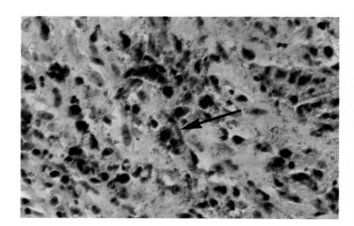

Fig. 8.2. **Histiocytosis X.**
Eosinophilic granuloma.
Same case as in *Fig.* 8.1.
Scattered Charcot–Leyden
crystals are present. The
crystal is typically fusiform
with tapered ends.
(PTAH × 480.)

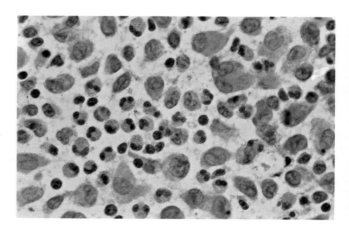

Fig. 8.3. **Histiocytosis X.**
Eosinophilic granuloma.
Same case as in *Figs.* 8.1 and
8.2. Smear showing an
admixture of histiocytes and
eosinophils. The histiocytes
are predominantly juvenile,
with large open nuclei. One
of the histiocytes is
binucleate. (HE × 480.)

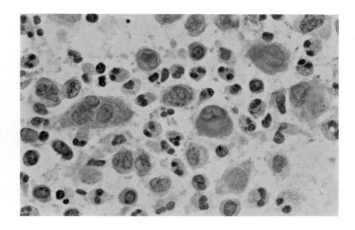

Fig. 8.4. **Histiocytosis X.**
Eosinophilic granuloma.
Same case as in *Figs.* 8.1–3.
Smear showing histiocytes
and eosinophils. One of the
histiocytes is multinucleate.
The histiocytes are juvenile
forms with open
uncondensed nuclei—
compare with small
condensed nucleus of a
senescent foamy histiocyte
(*Fig.* 8.6). (HE × 480.)

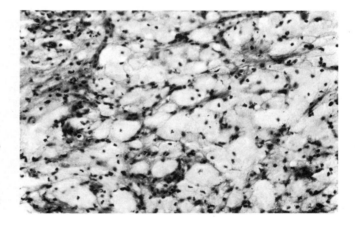

Fig. 8.5. **Histiocytosis X.**
Hand–Christian–Schüller
disease. Histology shows a
xanthomatous 'foam-celled'
histiocytic proliferate;
elsewhere occasional foci
showed less mature
histiocytes and eosinophils.
(HE × 192.)

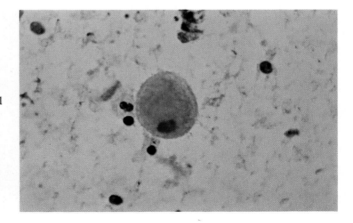

Fig. 8.6. **Histiocytosis X.**
Hand–Christian–Schüller
disease. Same case as in *Fig.*
8.5. Smear showing a typical
foam cell, a mature
histiocyte with condensed
nucleus and lipid
accumulation in its bloated
cytoplasm. A senile bilobed
eosinophil is seen to the left
of the foam cell, its granules
no longer identifiable.
(HE × 480.)

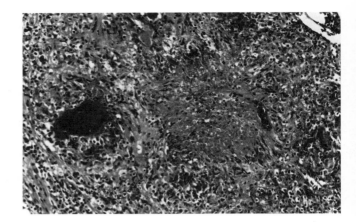

Fig. 8.7. **Tuberculosis.**
Histology of epithelioid
granuloma with central
caseation; a Langhans-type
giant-cell is present.
(HE × 192.)

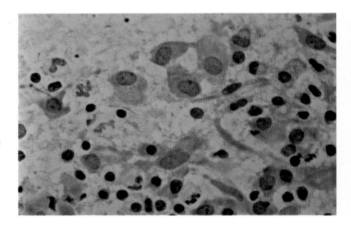

Fig. 8.8. **Tuberculosis.**
Same case as in *Fig.* 8.7.
Smear showing numerous
histiocytes, many of juvenile
type with large open nuclei.
Also included are several
fusiform fibrocytes,
lymphocytes and
polymorphonuclear
leucocytes. (HE × 480.)

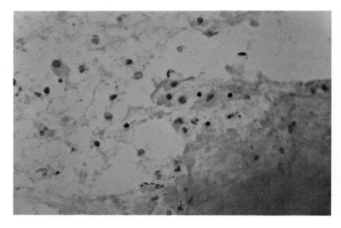

Fig. 8.9. **Tuberculosis.**
Same case as in *Figs.* 8.7 and
8.8. A low-power view of
the smear, to show part of
the amorphous debris
derived from the areas of
caseous necrosis. Scattered
histiocytes, fibrocytes,
lymphocytes and
polymorphs adjoin the
debris. (HE × 192.)

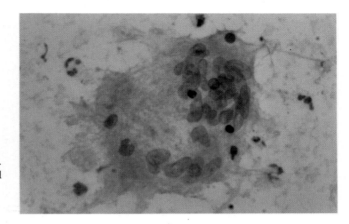

Fig. 8.10. **Tuberculosis.** Same case as in *Figs.* 8.7–9. Smear showing a Langhans-type multinucleate giant cell and several polymorphonuclear leucocytes. (HE × 480.)

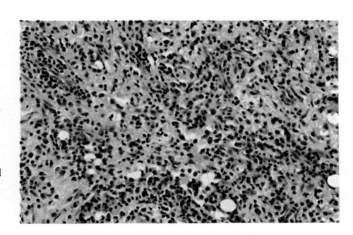

Fig. 8.11. **Chronic osteomyelitis.** Brodie's abscess. Histology is that of a non-specific chronic inflammatory reaction, containing an intimate admixture of lymphocytes, plasma cells, histiocytes and granulocytes. The relative proportions of these cells vary from case to case. (HE × 192.)

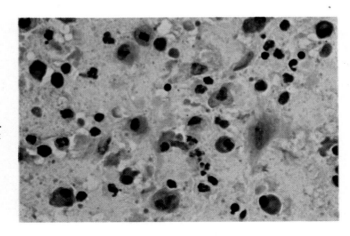

Fig. 8.12. **Chronic osteomyelitis.** Brodie's abscess. Same case as in *Fig.* 8.11. Smear showing a great variety of inflammatory cells—histiocytes, plasma cells, polymorphonuclear leucocytes, lymphocytes. Eosinophils may also be present in some cases. (HE × 480.)

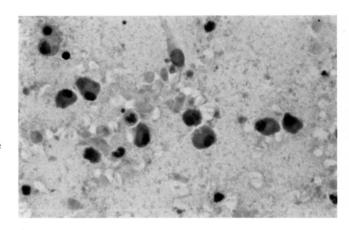

Fig. 8.13. **Chronic osteomyelitis.** Brodie's abscess. Same case as in *Figs.* 8.11 and 8.12. Part of smear showing preponderance of plasma cells. Rarely, chronic osteomyelitis may show a superabundance of plasma cells, the so-called 'pseudomyeloma'. In such a case the plasma cells are all mature, show no mitoses or nuclear pleomorphism as in plasma-cell myeloma (compare with *Fig.* 6.34, Chapter 6). (HE × 480.)

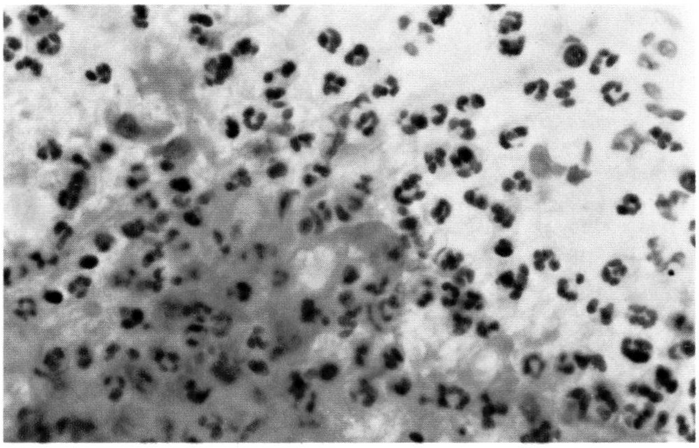

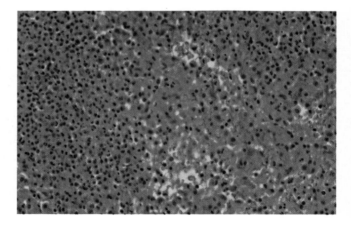

Fig. 8.14. **Acute osteomyelitis.** Smear from a needle aspiration biopsy, showing an acute inflammatory exudate, almost exclusively of polymorphonuclear leucocytes. (HE × 480.)

Fig. 8.15. **Subacute osteomyelitis.** Histological field showing small abscesses. Elsewhere the lesion showed granulation tissue with diffuse histiocytic proliferation and interspersed polymorphs. (HE × 192.)

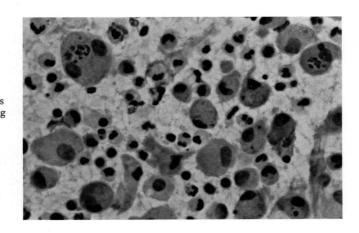

Fig. 8.16. **Subacute osteomyelitis.** Same case as in *Fig.* 8.15. Smear showing abundant histiocytes with scattered polymorphonuclear leucocytes. The histiocytes contain ingested pus cells and nuclear debris. Compare with eosinophilic granuloma (*Figs.* 8.3 and 8.4). (HE × 480.)

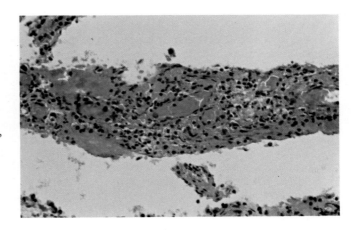

Fig. 8.17. **Subacute osteomyelitis.** Another case. Histology of drill core, showing hyperaemic tissue with scattered polymorphs. Compare with the smears (*Fig.* 8.18), which makes the diagnosis of infection even more explicit. (HE × 192.)

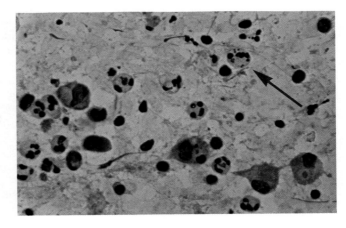

Fig. 8.18. **Subacute osteomyelitis.** Same case as in *Fig.* 8.17. Smear showing admixture of histiocytes—containing ingested polymorphs and nuclear debris—and polymorphonuclear leucocytes. The polymorph arrowed contains numerous cocci. (HE × 192.)

One example of this histological/cytological pattern will be given herein. The patient presented at the unusual age of 58 with a destructive lesion in the right tibia, whose nature could not be surmised radiologically. Histology showed extensive xanthomatous areas (*Fig.* 8.5) in addition to a few active histiocytic/eosinophilic foci. Cytological smears (*Fig.* 8.6) showed abundant foamy histiocytes. A diagnosis of eosinophilic granuloma was made. During the course of the following year, many other bones were involved and the patient developed diabetes insipidus, so that an ultimate diagnosis of Hand–Christian–Schüller disease was established.

TUBERCULOSIS

The typical histology of tuberculosis (*Fig.* 8.7) is well recognized: a histiocytic or 'epithelioid' granuloma showing follicular aggregates of histiocytes, with a tendency to central caseous necrosis and marginal collections of lymphocytes. Langhans-type multinucleate giant-cells are frequently present in the epithelioid tubercles. The extent of the caseous necrosis varies from case to case, and may be confluent or extensive. The degree of lymphocytic infiltration is variable likewise. Some superimposed infiltration by polymorphonuclear leucocytes may also be present.

These features are reflected in smears from osseous tuberculosis (*Figs.* 8.8–10). The caseous component is seen as focal collections of amorphous eosinophilic debris (*Fig.* 8.9) in which acid-alcohol-fast bacilli may occasionally be found. The histiocytes are clearly identifiable and show various stages of maturity. Scattered Langhans-type multinucleate giant-cells are usually present (*Fig.* 8.10), although they are not particularly frequent. There are fair numbers of lymphocytes, fibroblasts and scattered, often degenerate, polymorphonuclear leucocytes. Plasma cells are absent or, at best, extremely scanty.

A firm cytological diagnosis of tuberculosis cannot be made, unless acid-alcohol-fast bacilli are identified. The cytological diagnosis must be of a histiocytic granuloma, presumably tuberculosis.

CHRONIC OSTEOMYELITIS

As a diagnostic problem in orthopaedic practice, chronic osteomyelitis usually presents as a Brodie's abscess which is seen histologically (*Fig.* 8.11) as a focus of non-specific chronic inflammatory reaction in which there is a polymorphic infiltrate by plasma cells, lymphocytes, histiocytes, polymorphonuclear leucocytes and sometimes eosinophils. Bacteria may sometimes be identifiable.

Cytological smears (*Figs.* 8.12 and 8.13) from such a lesion fully reflect the cellular composition of the chronic inflammation: they show frequent plasma cells, fair numbers of lymphocytes, as well as histiocytes and polymorphonuclear leucocytes. This cytological picture is basically that of a non-specific chronic inflammatory exudate, so that in the absence of identifiable organisms an infective basis can only be inferred.

Rarely, in chronic osteomyelitis the plasma cells may overwhelmingly outnumber the other inflammatory cells, so that a fallacious diagnosis of myeloma may be entertained. In such cases, both in the histological sections and the cytological smears, the plasma cells are of normal morphology, are associated with Russell bodies; scattered lymphocytes, histiocytes and polymorphonuclear leucocytes are found; mitoses are absent.

ACUTE AND SUBACUTE OSTEOMYELITIS

From time to time cases present with osteolytic lesions in bone due to acute or subacute osteomyelitis in which there are no obvious clinical indications of infection, so that a malignant tumour such as 'malignant round-cell tumour' may be suspected. Some, but by no means all, such cases may be due to modification of the infective process by inadequate or incidental antibiotic treatment. Three such cases are presented below.

Case 1. A 2-month-old female infant was noticed to be reluctant to move her left arm, the shoulder was swollen and apparently caused pain on passive movement. The swelling appeared to be 'non-inflamed' and there was no pyrexia. X-rays showed patchy destruction of the upper humeral metaphysis and there was evidence of epiphysial detachment which was ascribed to birth injury. The presumptive diagnosis was of metastatic neuroblastoma, with low-grade infection as the alternative. A needle aspiration of the humeral lesion was performed. Smears (*Fig.* 8.14) showed a polymorphonuclear leucocytic exudate, establishing the diagnosis of acute osteomyelitis. Cultures of the aspirate yielded *Escherichia coli*.

Case 2. A man aged 25 presented with a history of pain in the left flank for about 3 weeks and a tender swelling was noticed over the left iliac crest. He had had no pyrexia at any time. X-rays showed an extensive area of osteolysis with patchy sclerosis in the ilium, interpreted as being suspicious of malignancy, possibly 'malignant round-cell tumour', perhaps even osteosarcoma. At surgical exploration, granulation tissue was found and a small amount of pus exuded.

Histologically (*Fig.* 8.15) there was a subacute inflammatory reaction with very abundant histiocytes interspersed with polymorphonuclear leucocytes; scattered focal micro-abscesses were present, full of degenerate or dead polymorphs.

Cytologically (*Fig.* 8.16), the smears are characteristic of a subacute inflammatory reaction. There are abundant histiocytes, some containing ingested pus cells, as well as many polymorphonuclear leucocytes. No bacteria were identified and cultures from the wound proved negative. The smears differ from those of Histiocytosis X in the absence of eosinophils and the abundance of polymorphs; they differ from those of tuberculosis in the absence of Langhans-type multinucleate giant cells and caseous debris, and in the abundance of polymorphonuclear leucocytes.

Case 3. A 12-year-old boy gave a 3-week history of pain and swelling in the left shoulder, followed by pain in the right knee and left ankle. He was afebrile, the WBC was normal and the ESR was raised. He had received antibiotic treatment elsewhere. X-rays of the proximal humerus, distal tibia and distal femur were thought to show changes suspicious of neoplasia. The lesions were therefore biopsied. Both the histology (*Fig.*8.17) and the cytology (*Fig.* 8.18) showed a subacute inflammatory reaction and Gram-positive cocci were identified. Staphylococci were cultured from the humeral lesion.

Chapter 9

Cystic Lesions of Bone

Whilst cytological examination is not of particular importance in the diagnosis of these conditions, an account of the cytological findings in their smears will be given here, if only to provide a comparison with the other conditions dealt with in this volume.

As with all bone lesions, the clinical features, radiological appearances and the operative findings will provide valuable guides to the pathologist in dealing with surgical material derived from cystic conditions. It is important to bear in mind that the actual amount of tissue that can be scraped or otherwise removed from cystic lesions is normally scanty in comparison with their actual size. The fluid content of the cyst should always give a good clue to its nature, but it is surprising how rarely this is specified in the surgical notes. The fluid present should be blood in aneurysmal bone cyst and, in uncomplicated cases, clear or straw-coloured fluid in simple bone cyst, mucoid fluid in intra-osseous ganglion and osteoarthritic cyst and pearly pultaceous material in epidermal cyst.

ANEURYSMAL BONE CYST

Aneurysmal bone cyst (*Fig.* 9.1) is characterized by a wide meshwork of cavernous blood-vascular spaces of variable dimensions, the septa of which are formed by fibro-cellular tissue with abundant osteoclasts; osteoblasts and osteoid matrix are also frequently present.

Cytological smears (*Fig.* 9.2) from the walls or septa of an aneurysmal bone cyst will be heavily bloodstained and will contain fusiform and rounded cells similar to those seen in non-ossifying fibroma, together with fairly abundant osteoclasts and a scattering of osteoblasts. The precise proportions of these cells will, of course, depend on their acutal numbers in the tissue sampled. There is nothing specific or diagnostic in such smears and aneurysmal bone cyst cannot be diagnosed from cytological smears alone. Predominantly fibrocellular smears from aneurysmal bone cyst may not be unlike those from non-ossifying fibroma; predominantly osteoclastic smears may simulate such giant-celled lesions as non-ossifying fibroma and giant-cell tumour.

SIMPLE BONE CYST

Simple bone cyst (*Fig.* 9.3) is lined by a relatively thin layer of fibrocellular tissue. Patchy osteoid formation with associated osteoblasts may be found in this tissue and scattered osteoclasts may also be present. In some cases loosely pedunculated coral-like formations (*Fig.* 9.4) may develop within the cyst, apparently after coagulation of blood, fibrin and proteinaceous sediment. This coagulum is flocculent and becomes partly or wholly calcified; it is gradually vascularized from

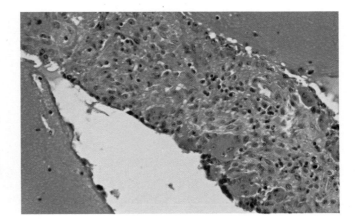

Fig. 9.1. **Aneurysmal bone cyst.** Histology of septum, with cavernous blood-containing spaces on either side. The septum is formed by rounded and fusiform cells, with osteoclasts tending to line the septal margin. (HE × 192.)

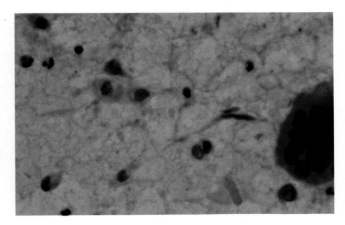

Fig. 9.2. **Aneurysmal bone cyst.** Same case as in *Fig.* 9.1. Smear showing part of an osteoclast and scattered rounded and fusiform ('fibro-histiocytic') cells. The smears faithfully reflect the cellular make-up of the lesional tissue in aneurysmal bone cyst, but a diagnosis of aneurysmal bone cyst cannot be made on the cytological findings. (HE × 480.)

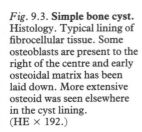

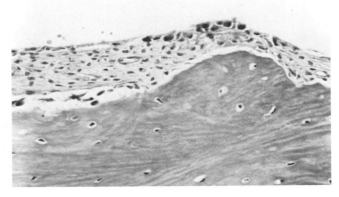

Fig. 9.3. **Simple bone cyst.** Histology. Typical lining of fibrocellular tissue. Some osteoblasts are present to the right of the centre and early osteoidal matrix has been laid down. More extensive osteoid was seen elsewhere in the cyst lining. (HE × 192.)

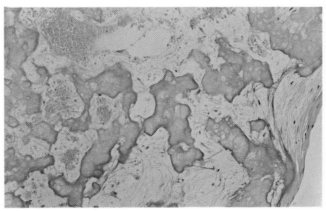

Fig. 9.4. **Simple bone cyst.**
Same case as in *Fig*. 9.3.
Histology of intra-cystic
structure. Floccules of
calcified coagulum with
early vascularization of the
intervening spaces.
Eventually actual
ossification occurs around
the floccules. (HE × 120.)

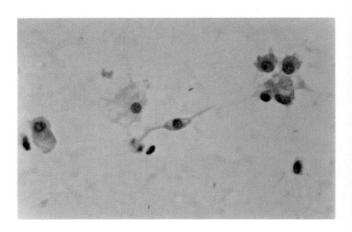

Fig. 9.5. **Simple bone cyst.**
Same case as in *Figs*. 9.3 and
9.4. Smear from cyst lining,
showing predominantly
mononuclear cells; fusiform
cell is also included. The
mononuclear cells are
essentially similar to those
seen in non-ossifying
fibroma. (HE × 480.)

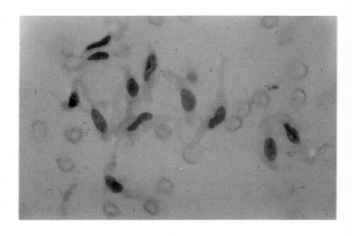

Fig. 9.6. **Simple bone cyst.**
Another case. Smear from
cyst lining, in this instance
predominantly fibrocytic.
Smears from simple bone
cyst reflect the cellular
composition of the cyst wall,
but a diagnosis of simple
bone cyst cannot be made on
the cytological findings.
(HE × 480.)

Fig. 9.7. **Osteoarthritic bone cyst.** Biopsy of 'solid' mass, suspected at operation of being a fibrosarcoma or chondrosarcoma. Representative histology, showing irregular strands of fibrinoid material (staining blue here, but red with eosin), metachromatic (purple-red) mucoid fluid, and fragments of necrotic cartilage (pale purple-blue), irregularly admixed. No viable tissue present. (Taylor's blue × 120.)

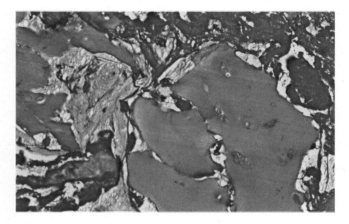

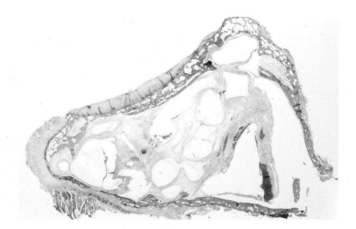

Fig. 9.8. **Intra-osseous ganglion.** Mounted section to show multilocular cyst in head of fibula. (HE × 2·4.)

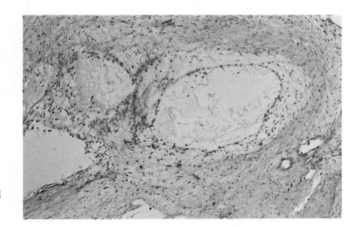

Fig. 9.9. **Intra-osseous ganglion.** Same case as in *Fig.* 9.8. Histology of smaller, developing loculi, showing loose fibro-myxoid tissue in the cyst wall. (HE × 48.)

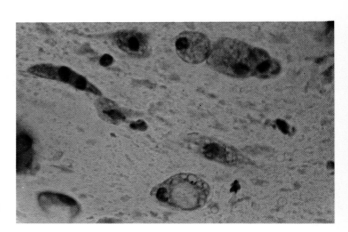

Fig. 9.10. **Intra-osseous ganglion.** Same case as in *Figs.* 9.8 and 9.9. Smear showing typical cells from myxomatous area; these have developed through metaplasia of fibroblastic cells. They have become rounded up and bloated through intracytoplasmic secretion of mucin. A similar picture can be seen with myxoid osteoarthritic cysts and 'ganglia' of the soft tissues. (HE × 480.)

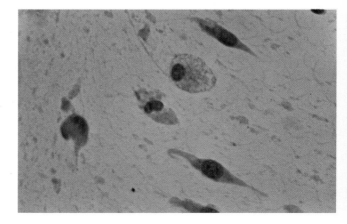

Fig. 9.11. **Intra-osseous ganglion.** Same case as in *Figs.* 9.8–10. Smear showing gradations between fusiform fibroblastic cells and bloated vacuolated myxomatous cells. The vacuolation is due to secretion of connective tissue mucin. The fusiform cell at top shows early vacuolation of its cytoplasm. (HE × 480.)

the adjoining wall and undergoes subsequent ossification. Such intra-cystic bodies have sometimes been misconstrued as 'cementomas' of the long bones (Friedman and Goldman, 1969).

Smears from the lining of a simple bone cyst (*Figs.* 9.5 and 9.6) yield a scanty population of rounded or fusiform cells of the type seen in non-ossifying fibromas; one or the other type of cell may predominate according to the actual composition of the sampled tissue. Random osteoclasts and osteoblasts may be found. There is nothing specific or diagnostic in these smears; they merely reflect the cellular composition of the cyst lining. Eosinophilic or calcific debris may be found in the smears in cases containing calcifying coagulum in the cyst cavity.

OSTEOARTHRITIC BONE CYST

Subarticular cysts are commonplace in osteoarthritis. They are usually a centimetre or less in diameter. Not all 'cysts' demonstrable radiologically are actually cystic; some may be filled by myxoid and fibromyxoid connective tissue. However, even such solid lesions may contain cartilaginous or osseous debris in their substance. Such debris is shed from the abraded articular surface into the synovial fluid and thence forced into the subarticular cysts by the intra-articular pressure. Their presence in solid fibromyxoid subarticular lesions indicates that at one time these must have been cystic and in communication with the joint cavity. Because they contain bony–cartilaginous debris, osteoarthritic cysts have sometimes been called 'detritus cysts' (Jaffe, 1972). Similar subarticular cysts may also occur in rheumatoid arthritis.

Occasionally, exceptionally large osteoarthritic cysts occur and may cause diagnostic problems. We have come across several instances of this phenomenon and here give one example. A 57-year-old man was found to have a para-articular mass at the hip, fixed to and involving the acetabular margin. Clinically a fibrosarcoma or chondrosarcoma was suspected; at surgical exploration a solid myxoid mass was found deeply extending into the acetabular margin. Biopsy showed the mass to consist of an extensive meshwork of fibrinous material (*Fig.* 9.7) with metachromatic mucin in the interstices and containing abundant cartilaginous and some osseous debris. A diagnosis of osteoarthritic cyst was made and was confirmed by subsequent excision of the lesion.

Not surprisingly, cytological smears from this particular osteoarthritic cyst were acellular, showing only fibrinous debris and metachromatic mucin. Smears from the partly or wholly solid fibromyxoid subarticular cysts yield fibrous and myxoid cells similar to those found in intra-osseous ganglia (*see below*).

INTRA-OSSEOUS GANGLION (JUXTA-ARTICULAR BONE CYST)

These cysts (*Figs.* 9.8 and 9.9) contain mucoid fluid just like the common 'ganglia' of the extra-osseous connective tissues and are similarly lined by fibrous or fibromyxoid tissue. In the examples recorded in this Registry there has been no demonstrable communication with the adjoining joint cavity and, unlike the osteoarthritic cysts, they do not contain bony/cartilaginous detritus.

Smears from their walls (*Figs.* 9.10 and 9.11) show fibrocytic and myxoid cells of benign cytomorphology.

INTRA-OSSEOUS EPIDERMAL CYST

Epidermal cysts may occasionally be found in bones, especially in the terminal phalanges of the fingers. They do not give rise to any diagnostic problems and their macroscopic appearance is readily recognizable. One example was smeared here and, as expected, showed the typical cornified squames of the epidermal cuticle.

References

Friedman N.B. and Goldman R.L. (1969) Cementoma of long bones: an extragnathic odontogenic tumor. *Clin. Orthop.* **67**, 243.

Jaffe H.L. (1972) *Metabolic, Degenerative and Inflammatory Diseases of Bones and Joints.* Philadelphia, Lea & Febiger, p. 750.

Chapter 10

Some Rare and Unusual Tumours of Bone

A variety of rare and unusual bone tumours exist, most of which we have either not recorded in this Registry or else have not studied cytologically. It is not our intention to give a full list of these tumours, but they include liposarcoma, angiosarcoma, adamantinoma of the long bones, glomus tumour, malignant fibrous histiocytoma and leiomyosarcoma.

We have had no experience of angiosarcoma of bone, nor have we had occasion to study the cytology of any soft-tissue angiosarcomas. Likewise, we have had no smears from glomus tumour or adamantinoma of the long bones. We suspect that there might be considerable difficulty in the cytological differentiation of adamantinoma of the long bones from metastatic carcinoma.

LIPOSARCOMA

Liposarcoma in bone would not differ in its histological and cytological features from the usual extra-osseous example of that tumour, illustrations of which are given in *Figs.* 10.1–3. Alkaline phosphatase is present in the malignant lipoblasts which also contain abundant lipid. The possible problem in the cytological differentiation of liposarcoma from osteosarcoma has already been referred to in Chapter 2.

MALIGNANT FIBROUS HISTIOCYTOMA

Malignant fibrous histiocytoma has only recently been reported in bone (Feldman and Norman, 1972; Huvos, 1976; Dahlin et al., 1977). We have recently seen a typical example (*Fig.* 10.4) in this laboratory, unfortunately with referred histological material without any cytological smears. We do not, therefore, know whether the cytology of malignant fibrous histiocytoma differs significantly from that of fibrosarcoma. Several problems will arise from this new entity among bone tumours. There is the danger that malignant fibrous histiocytoma will be increasingly diagnosed whenever a pleomorphic unspecified sarcoma presents in bone, thus exaggerating its true incidence; we feel this is already happening with many soft-tissue sarcomas. The existing statistics on fibrosarcoma of bone are already partly vitiated by the inclusion of an unspecified number of fibroblastic osteosarcomas; they must be further bedevilled by the probability, based on the data of Dahlin et al. (1977), that a further 10 % might have been examples of malignant fibrous histiocytoma.

LEIOMYOSARCOMA

Only a few reports of leiomyosarcoma of bone have been recorded in the literature (Evans and Sanerkin, 1965; Overgaard et al., 1977). We have recently seen two

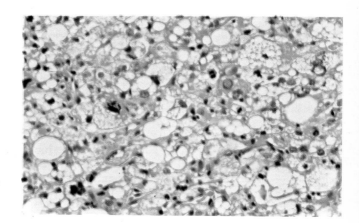

Fig. 10.1. **Liposarcoma.**
Example from the soft
tissues. Histology typical of
pleomorphic liposarcoma.
(HE × 192.)

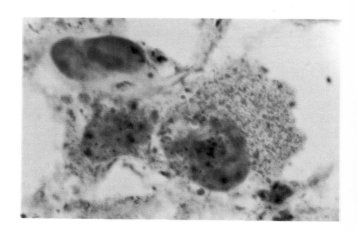

Fig. 10.2. **Liposarcoma.**
Same case as in *Fig.* 10.1.
Tumour cells containing
lipid. (Oil Red O × 480.)

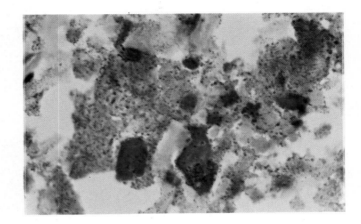

Fig. 10.3. **Liposarcoma.**
Same case as in *Figs.* 10.1
and 10.2. Tumour cells
containing alkaline
phosphatase. (Alkaline
phosphatase
preparation × 480.)

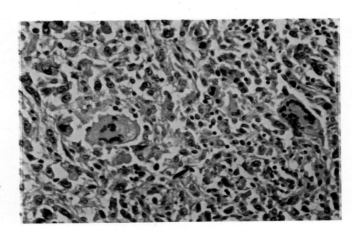

Fig. 10.4. **Malignant
fibrous histiocytoma.**
Histology. Pleomorphic
predominantly histiocytic
part of tumour, with
scattered giant tumour cells.
Other parts showed a
storiform spindle-celled
tumour. (HE × 192.)

Fig. 10.5. **Leiomyo-sarcoma.** Histological section through longitudinal and transverse bundles of tumour cells. Cells sectioned longitudinally show considerably elongated cytoplasmic prolongations; one of the cells has two nuclei in tandem (arrowed). Cells sectioned transversely show scanty nuclei; most of the cells have been cut through their cytoplasmic prolongations. (HE × 192.)

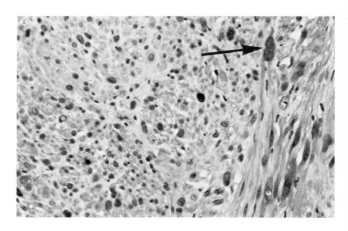

Fig. 10.6. **Leiomyo-sarcoma.** Similar field as in *Fig.* 10.5, stained for reticulin. In longitudinal section, the reticulin is arranged in converging tram-lines. In transverse section, a distinct pericellular honeycomb pattern is seen. (Reticulin × 192.)

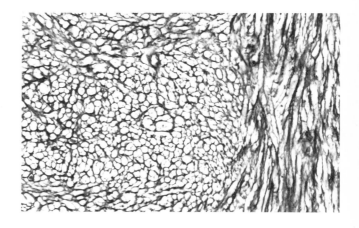

Fig. 10.7. **Leiomyo-sarcoma.** Same case as in *Figs.* 10.5 and 10.6. Myofibrils are demonstrable in many of the tumour cells. (PTAH × 192.)

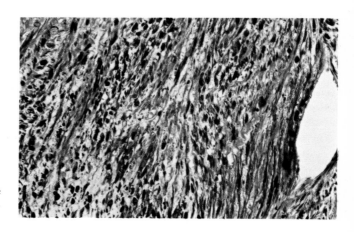

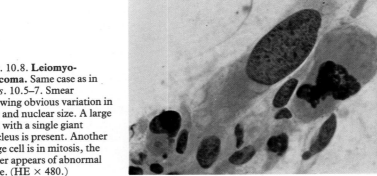

Fig. 10.8. **Leiomyosarcoma.** Same case as in *Figs*. 10.5–7. Smear showing obvious variation in cell and nuclear size. A large cell with a single giant nucleus is present. Another large cell is in mitosis, the latter appears of abnormal type. (HE × 480.)

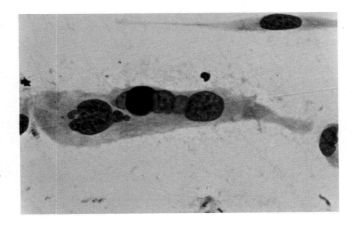

Fig. 10.9. **Leiomyosarcoma.** Same case as in *Figs*. 10.5–8. Elongated giant tumour cell with multiple nuclei. The nuclei are arranged in a beaded row; the nuclear size and intensity of staining variable. A small tumour cell (*top right*) shows a cigar-shaped nucleus and greatly elongated cytoplasm. (HE × 480.)

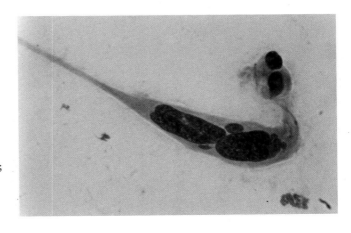

Fig. 10.10. **Leiomyosarcoma.** Same case as in *Figs*. 10.5–9. Giant multinucleate tumour cell with elongated cytoplasm. Larger nuclei are in tandem; several tiny nuclei are also present, including a cluster at the right end. (HE × 480.)

additional examples. In the second of these, we had access to fresh tumour tissue and were able to study its cytology. The patient was a woman aged 61 with a destructive lesion in the upper end of the right tibia and no other demonstrable tumours elsewhere in the body. Histologically (*Fig.* 10.5) this is a spindle-cell sarcoma with elongated cells having fairly abundant eosinophilic cytoplasm and ovoid or elongated nuclei. Binucleate and multinucleate cells are fairly frequent and the nuclei in such cells are arranged in tandem or in series along the long axis of the cell. The reticulin stroma (*Fig.* 10.6) is pericellular, appearing as converging tramlines in longitudinal section and as a honeycomb pattern in cross section. Myofibrils are demonstrable in PTAH sections (*Fig.* 10.7) and by electron microscopy. Glycogen is also present in some of the tumour cells.

Smears show elongated cells with fairly abundant cytoplasm and considerable variation in cell and nuclear size (*Figs.* 10.8–10). Many binucleate cells are seen, the nuclei being in tandem and rather widely separated from one another. Multinucleate tumour cells (*Figs.* 10.9 and 10.10) show the nuclei arranged in beaded manner along the long axis of the cell. In addition to the larger nuclei, numerous clusters of tiny nuclei may be seen in such cells. No acid or alkaline phosphatase is demonstrable in the tumour cells. We had hoped to demonstrate myofibrils in the smeared cells, but PTAH failed to show these in the smears; cryostat sections and paraffin sections, *after rapid fixation in formol-saline*, also failed to show PTAH-positive myofibrils. For comparison, smears and cryostat sections were prepared from human uterine muscle, and these too failed to show myofibrils; likewise, paraffin sections after rapid fixation in formol-saline proved negative. Demonstration of myofibrils with PTAH was only possible after overnight fixation, in both the uterine muscle and in the tumour in question.

References
Dahlin D.C., Unni K.K. and Matsuno T. (1977) Malignant (fibrous) histiocytoma of bone—fact or fancy? *Cancer 39*, 1508.
Evans D.M.D. and Sanerkin N.G. (1965) Primary leiomyosarcoma of bone. *J. Pathol. Bact. 90*, 348.
Feldman F. and Norman D. (1972) Intra- and extraosseous malignant histiocytoma (malignant fibrous xanthoma). *Radiology 104*, 497.
Huvos A.G. (1976) Primary malignant fibrous histiocytoma of bone: clinicopathologic study of 18 patients. *N.Y. State J. Med. 76*, 552.
Overgaard J., Frederiksen P., Helmig O. et al. (1977) Primary leiomyosarcoma of bone. *Cancer 39*, 1664.

Technical Methods

The practical details of the various enzyme cytochemistry techniques and routine staining procedures, as applied to cytological smears in this Laboratory, are set out in this appendix.

It is our practice to use unfixed air-dried smears for enzyme cytochemistry. For all routine staining procedures, except Giemsa and Oil Red O, we prefer fixation of air-dried smears in cold acetone, but methanol at room temperature may be used as an alternative. For Giemsa the air-dried smears are fixed in methanol and for Oil Red O they are fixed in 10 % neutral formol saline.

Smears stained with routine stains are mounted in a synthetic resin medium, such as XAM or DPX. Smears stained with Oil Red O and all enzyme cytochemistry preparations are mounted in PVP or glycerin jelly. Details for the preparation of PVP (Burstone, 1957) are given below:

Dissolve 50 g polyvinyl pyrrolidone (mol. wt. approx. 44 000) in 50 ml distilled water. Stand overnight. Add 2 ml glycerol and a crystal of thymol and stir. Neutralize with sodium hydroxide solution till pH is approximately 8·0.

The staining methods are essentially those in the references quoted, but with minor modifications that we have found convenient, although we do not claim any general advantage from these slight variations.

1. TECHNIQUES FOR ENZYME CYTOCHEMISTRY

For economy of substrate the following procedure is recommended in all cases in enzyme cytochemistry and histochemistry (Jeffree, 1969b):

A 7-inch length of 1½-inch polythene tubing is folded in half and stood with the folded end in a Coplin jar. 10 ml of the staining solution is poured into one open end and the smeared slide is incubated in this. Using this method, one slide, or two slides placed back-to-back, can be stained in 10 ml of solution instead of the 50 ml required for a Coplin jar.

Alkaline phosphatase (Burstone, 1958a)

Stock solutions:

0·2 M Tris buffer pH 8·3:

Tris (hydroxymethyl) aminomethane	24·2 g
N/1 hydrochloric acid	100 ml

Make up to 1 litre with distilled water.

Naphthol AS–TR phosphate solution:

40 mg/ml naphthol AS–TR phosphoric acid in dimethyl formamide.

Preparation of incubating medium:

0·2 M Tris buffer pH 8·3	10 ml
Naphthol AS–TR phosphate solution	0·02 ml
Fast Red Salt TR	6–10 mg

Method:

Use unfixed smears, air-dried.
1. Incubate at 37 °C, 20 minutes.
2. Wash in running water.
3. Harris's haematoxylin, 2–3 minutes.
4. Wash in running water till blue.
5. Mount in PVP or glycerin jelly.

Site of alkaline phosphatase activity—red.

Acid phosphatase (Burstone, 1958b)

Stock solutions:

0·1 M Acetate buffer pH 5·4:

N/1 sodium acetate	86 ml
N/1 acetic acid	14 ml
Distilled water	900 ml

Naphthol AS–TR phosphate solution:

40 mg/ml naphthol AS–TR phosphoric acid in dimethyl formamide.

Preparation of incubating medium:

0·1 M acetate buffer pH 5·4	10 ml
Naphthol AS–TR phosphate solution	0·02 ml
Fast Bordeaux OL	6–10 mg

Note: Fast Bordeaux OL is no longer commercially available. We suggest Fast Ponceau Salt L (C.I. 37151) as a suitable readily obtainable alternative (from G.T. Gurr, Hopkin and Williams). The commonly recommended alternative, Fast Red Violet LB Salt, can be difficult to obtain in this country.

Method:

Use unfixed smears, air-dried.
1. Incubate at 37 °C, 20 minutes.
2. Wash in running water.
3. Harris's haematoxylin, 2–3 minutes.
4. Wash in running water till blue.
5. Mount in PVP or glycerin jelly.

Site of acid phosphatase activity—red.

'Neutral' phosphatase (Jeffree, 1970)

Stock solutions:

Veronal Acetate Buffer pH 7·5:

Sodium acetate (trihydrate)	9·714 g
Barbitone sodium	14·714 g

Make up to 500 ml with distilled water
Take 50 ml of this solution, add 49 ml N/10 hydrochloric acid
Dilute to 250 ml with distilled water to give a final pH of 7·5

Naphthol AS–TR phosphate solution:

40 mg/ml naphthol AS–TR phosphoric acid in dimethyl formamide

Preparation of incubating media:
    A. Veronal acetate buffer pH 7·5   10 ml
        Naphthol AS–TR phosphate solution   0·02 ml
        Fast Red Salt TR   6–10 mg
    B. Veronal acetate buffer pH 7·5   10 ml
        Naphthol AS–TR phosphate solution   0·02 ml
        Fast Bordeaux OL   6–10 mg

Note: Fast Bordeaux OL is no longer commercially available. We suggest Fast Ponceau Salt L (C.I. 37151) as a suitable readily available alternative (from G.T. Gurr, Hopkin and Williams). The commonly recommended alternative, Fast Red Violet LB Salt, can be difficult to obtain in this country.

Method:
    Two unfixed smears, air-dried, are required.
    1. Incubate one smear in each of the incubating media (A and B above) at 37 °C for 20 minutes.
    2. Wash in running water.
    3. Harris's haematoxylin, 2–3 minutes.
    4. Wash in running water till blue.
    5. Mount in PVP or glycerin jelly.

A staining reaction present in A only indicates the presence of 'neutral' phosphatase.

A staining reaction present in both A and B indicates the presence of alkaline phosphatase.

Beta-glucuronidase (Jeffree, 1969a)

Stock solution:
    0·1 M Acetate buffer pH 5·0:
        N/1 sodium acetate   140 ml
        N/1 acetic acid   60 ml
        Distilled water   800 ml
    For use dilute 50 : 50 with distilled water

Preparation of incubating medium:
    Dissolve 2–3 mg naphthol AS–BI glucuronide in 0·2 ml sodium bicarbonate at 37 °C
    Add: 0·1 M acetate buffer pH 5·0   10 ml
        Fast Bordeaux OL   6–10 mg
    (This mixture will keep for several months deep-frozen in 10 ml aliquots.)

    Note: Fast Bordeaux OL is no longer commercially available. We suggest Fast Ponceau Salt L (C.I. 37151) as a suitable readily obtainable alternative (from G.T. Gurr, Hopkin and Williams). The commonly recommended alternative, Fast Red Violet LB Salt, can be difficult to obtain in this country.

Method:
    Use unfixed smears, air-dried.
    1. Incubate at 37 °C for 1 hour.
    2. Wash in running water.
    3. Harris's haematoxylin, 2–3 minutes.
    4. Wash in running water till blue.

5. Mount in PVP or glycerin jelly.
Site of beta-glucuronidase activity—red.

Monoamine oxidase (Glenner et al., 1957)
Stock solution:
  Phosphate buffer pH 7·6:
    0·06 M potassium dihydrogen orthophosphate   12 ml
    0·06 M disodium hydrogen orthophosphate   88 ml
Preparation of incubating medium:
    Tryptamine hydrochloride   25 mg
    Sodium sulphate   4 mg
    Nitro-blue tetrazolium   5 mg
    Phosphate buffer pH 7·6   5 ml
    Distilled water   15 ml
Method:
  Use unfixed smears, air-dried
    1. Incubate at 37 °C for 30–45 minutes.
    2. Wash in running water.
    3. Fix in neutral 10 % formol–saline for 24 hours.
    4. Counterstain in Mayer's carmalum.
    5. Rinse in running water.
    6. Mount in PVP or glycerin jelly.
Site of monoamine oxidase activity—blue-black.

Dopa-oxidase (tyrosinase) reaction (Laidlaw and Blackberg, 1932; Gomori, 1952)
Stock solution:
  Phosphate buffer pH 7·4:
    0·06 M potassium dihydrogen orthophosphate   20 ml
    0·06 M disodium hydrogen orthophosphate   80 ml
Preparation of incubating medium:
    0·1 % dihydroxyphenylalanine (DOPA) in phosphate buffer pH 7·4
Method:
  Use unfixed smears, air-dried.
    1. Incubate for 1 hour at 37 °C.
    2. Change to fresh incubating medium and leave at 37 °C for a further 2–3 hours.
    3. Wash in running water.
    4. Counterstain in Mayer's carmalum.
    5. Rinse in water.
    6. Mount in PVP or glycerin jelly.
DOPA-oxidase (tyrosinase) activity—dark brown granules.

2. ROUTINE STAINING PROCEDURES

Haematoxylin and eosin (Drury and Wallington, 1967)
Method:
    1. Fix smear in cold acetone, 2 minutes.
    2. Wash in running water.
    3. Harris's haematoxylin, 10 minutes.

4. Wash in running water till blue.
5. Differentiate in 1 % acid alcohol.
6. Wash in running water till blue.
7. 1 % aqueous eosin, 5 minutes.
8. Wash in running water.
9. Dehydrate, clear and mount in a synthetic resin medium.

Giemsa (Gurr, 1963)

Preparation of Giemsa stain:
Buffered water pH 6·8:

M/15 disodium hydrogen orthophosphate	50 ml
M/15 potassium dihydrogen orthophosphate	50 ml
Distilled water	400 ml

For use, dilute 10 drops of Gurr's Improved Giemsa Stain R66 with 10 ml buffered water and mix.

Method:
1. Fix smear in 100 % methanol, 2 minutes.
2. Stain in buffered Giemsa solution, 20–30 minutes.
3. Rinse in distilled water.
4. Allow to dry and mount in a synthetic medium.

Taylor's blue (Taylor and Jeffree, 1969)

Preparation of staining solution:
A. Stock solution of dye:

1:9, dimethyl methylene blue (Koch Light*)	0·5 g
Distilled water	100 ml

Stir mechanically for 30 minutes, then filter.
B. Buffer solution:

Sodium acetate (trihydrate)	9·714 g
Barbitone sodium	14·714 g

Make up to 500 ml with distilled water.
Take 50 ml of this solution, add 70 ml 0·1N hydrochloric acid.
Dilute to 250 ml with distilled water. This gives a final solution buffered to pH 6·12.

Working solution:

Taylor's blue	20 ml
Taylor's buffer	80 ml

(Alternatively, commercially prepared solutions may be obtained from Clin-Tech Ltd.†)

Method:
1. Fix smear in cold acetone, 2 minutes.
2. Wash in running water.
3. Buffered stain solution, 5 minutes.
4. Rinse in running water.
5. Pass rapidly through 50 % and 100 % dioxan (or acetone).
6. Rinse in 50:50 chloroform : xylene.
7. Clear in xylene and mount in a synthetic medium.

*Koch Light Laboratories Ltd, Colnbrook, SL3 0BZ, Buckinghamshire, England.
†Clin-Tech Ltd, 1–2 Faraday Way, Westminster Industrial Estate, London, SE18 5TR, England.

Periodic acid-Schiff (PAS) (McManus, 1946; modified by Pearse, 1968).
Method:
1. Fix smear in cold acetone, 2 minutes.
2. Wash in running water.
3. 2 % aqueous periodic acid, 5 minutes.
4. Wash in running water, 5 minutes.
5. Rinse in distilled water.
6. Schiff reagent, 10–20 minutes.
7. Rinse in distilled water.
8. Wash in running water, 10–20 minutes.
9. Harris's haematoxylin, 2–3 minutes.
10. Wash in running water till blue.
11. Dehydrate, clear and mount in a synthetic medium.
Glycogen, neutral mucin, glycoproteins—pink or purple red.

PAS–diastase
Method:
1. Fix smear in cold acetone, 2 minutes.
2. Wash in running water.
3. Treat with human saliva, or with a 0·1 % malt diastase in distilled water, freshly prepared, for 30 minutes at 37 °C.
4. Wash in running water, 5 minutes.
Subsequent steps as in 3–11 for PAS stain.
Glycogen–unstained.
Neutral mucin, glycoproteins—pink or purple red.

Oil Red O: (Barka and Anderson, 1963)
Preparation of Oil Red O solution:
1 % Oil Red O in 60 % triethyl phosphate.
Heat to 56 °C for 2–3 hours. Filter while hot, then cool.
Method:
1. Fix smear in 10 % neutral formol-saline, 5 minutes.
2. Wash in running water.
3. 60 % triethyl phosphate, 2–3 minutes.
4. Oil Red O solution, 20 minutes.
5. Rinse with 60 % triethyl phosphate.
6. Harris's haematoxylin, 2–3 minutes.
8. Wash in running water till blue.
9. Mount in PVP or glycerin jelly.
Neutral lipid—red.

Perl's Prussian Blue Reaction (Drury and Wallington, 1967)
Method:
1. Fix smear in cold acetone, 2 minutes.
2. Wash in running water.
3. Rinse in distilled water.
4. Transfer to a mixture of equal parts 2 % aqueous potassium ferrocyanide and 2 % hydrochloric acid, 20–30 minutes.
5. Wash in distilled water.
6. Counterstain in 1 % aqueous neutral red, 2–3 minutes.

7. Dehydrate, clear and mount in a synthetic medium.
Haemosiderin—blue.

Schmorl (Drury and Wallington, 1967)

Preparation of ferric–ferricyanide solution:
Take 4 ml fresh 1 % aqueous potassium ferricyanide, add 30 ml 1 % aqueous ferric chloride and an additional 6 ml distilled water.
This solution should be prepared just before use.
Method:
1. Fix smear in cold acetone, 2 minutes.
2. Wash in distilled water.
3. Treat with ferric–ferricyanide solution, 10 minutes.
4. Wash briefly in 1 % aqueous acetic acid.
5. Wash in running water.
6. Counterstain in 1 % aqueous neutral red, 2–3 minutes.
7. Rinse in water.
8. Dehydrate, clear and mount in a synthetic medium.
Reducing substances (e.g. melanin)—blue.

Masson–Fontana for melanin (Drury and Wallington, 1967)

Preparation of the silver solution:
Add strong ammonia drop-by-drop to 20 ml of 10 % silver nitrate until only a slight precipitate still remains, then add 20 ml of distilled water.
Method:
1. Fix smear in cold acetone, 2 minutes.
2. Wash well in distilled water.
3. Leave overnight in the silver solution in the dark in a closed jar.
4. Rinse well in distilled water.
5. Tone in 0·2 % aqueous gold chloride, 2–3 minutes.
6. Rinse in distilled water.
7. Fix in 5 % aqueous sodium thiosulphate, 2 minutes.
8. Wash in running water.
9. Counterstain in 1 % aqueous neutral red, 2–3 minutes.
10. Rinse in water.
11. Dehydrate, clear and mount in a synthetic medium.
Melanin—black.

References

Barka T. and Anderson P.J. (1963) *Histochemistry: Theory, Practice and Bibliography*. New York, Harper & Row.
Burstone M.S. (1957) Polyvinyl pyrrolidone as a mounting medium for stains for fat and for azo-dye procedures. *Am. J. Clin. Pathol. 28*, 429.
Burstone M.S. (1958a) Histochemical comparison of Naphthol AS-phosphates for the demonstration of phosphatases. *J. Natl. Cancer Inst. 20*, 601.
Burstone M.S. (1958b) Histochemical demonstration of acid phosphatase with Naphthol AS-phosphates. *J. Natl. Cancer Inst. 21*, 523.
Drury R.A.B. and Wallington E.A. (1967) *Carleton's Histological Technique*, 4th ed. London, Oxford University Press.
Glenner G.G., Burtner H.J. and Brown G.W. jun. (1957) The histochemical demonstration of monoamine oxidase activity by tetrazolium salts. *J. Histochem. Cytochem. 5*, 591.
Gomori G. (1952) *Microscopic Histochemistry: Principles and Practice*. Chicago, Ill., University of Chicago Press.
Gurr G.T. (1963) *Biological Staining Methods*, 7th ed. London, Gurr.

Jeffree G.M. (1969a) Demonstration of beta-glucuronidase with naphthol AS-BI-beta-D glucosiduronic acid by simultaneous coupling. *J. Microsc. (Oxf.)* **89**, 55.

Jeffree G.M. (1969b) A note on economy of substrate in enzyme histochemistry. *Histochem. J.* **1**, 278.

Jeffree G.M. (1970) The histochemical differentiation of various phosphatases in a population of osteoclasts by a simultaneous coupling method using different diazonium salts, with observations on the presence of inhibitors in stable diazonium salts. *Histochem. J.* **2**, 231.

Laidlaw G.F. and Blackberg S.N. (1932) Melanoma studies. II, A simple technique for the DOPA reaction. *Am. J. Pathol.* **8**, 491.

McManus J.F.A. (1946) Histological demonstration of mucin after periodic acid. *Nature (Lond.)* **158**, 202.

Pearse A.G.E. (1968) *Histochemistry: Theoretical and Applied*, 3rd ed., vol. 1. Boston, Little, Brown.

Taylor K.B. and Jeffree G.M. (1969) A new basic metachromatic dye, 1:9-Dimethyl Methylene Blue. *Histochem. J.* **1**, 199.

INDEX